"Dr. Tick's novel, integrated approach to the diagnosis and treatment of a wide variety of musculoskeletal disorders-specifically "RSI" is a must read for patients and health care providers alike. It represents a truly unique synthesis of mind, body and spirit; just what the doctor ordered for the new 21rst century medicine.""

W. Mark Erwin DC, PhD
Assistant Professor, Division of Orthopaedic Surgery, Spine Programme,
University of Toronto

"Dr. Tick's book, *Life Beyond Carpal Tunnel*, is a rich source of information, support, and healing resources for all that suffer from repetitive strain injuries or RSI. Her book covers a broad range of activities and exercises to prevent RSI as well as reducing the symptoms. For the sufferer, it gives them the support of knowing that this is a real condition and not in their head; and tools for healing. As our culture continues toward a culture of computers and repetitive movement jobs, RSI will increase the costs to us all. Dr. Tick's book is a must-read for anyone that works with repetitive movements and computers. It will protect them and support them in moving from pain to healing."

Steven Gurgevich, PhD
Tranceformation Works! (div. of Behavioral Medicine, Ltd.)
www.TheSelf-HypnosisDiet.com

"Human evolution has hit a brick wall. Today's information based work requires highly repetitive movements combined with static and awkward postures which have lead to an epidemic in soft tissue injuries such as Carpal Tunnel Syndrome. *Life Beyond the Carpal Tunnel* is a "Human User Manual". It is written with you in mind, in easy to understand language and is based on Dr. Tick's extensive experience in finding real world solutions to these evolutionary challenges".

Fraser McDonald
President, Humanomics Inc.
Ergonomics Intervention Specialist

"Dr. Tick has written a useful, comprehensive and empowering book on RSI. Every aspect of this condition is addressed in a way that equips patients with the tools they need to both connect with their physician and get better. Modalities such as IMS and good lifestyle habits (nutrition, sleep hygiene, work ergonomics, exercise) are key cornerstones for long-term healing."

Gordon Ko MD, CCFP(EM), FRCPC, FAAPMR, CIME, CMAS, N.MD
Director of the Physiatry Interventional Treatment Clinic at Sunnybrook Health Sciences Centre in Toronto, (Dept of Rehabilitation Medicine.) Medical director for the Canadian Centre for Integrative Medicine.

THE RSI CLINIC HANDBOOK

Life Beyond the Carpal Tunnel

Heather Tick

This book is not medical advice and the author does not dispense medical advice or prescribe the use of any technique for the treatment of injuries or illness. The purpose of this book is to provide information. Please consult a health care provider for specific information regarding any injury or condition.

None of the stories about patients in this book represent one person. They are composites of several people and the aim is to present some common scenarios which have been encountered in our clinic.

Printed in Canada
This is a Healing Weave Publication
FIN 17 08 07

Library and Archives Canada Cataloguing in Publication

Tick, Heather,
        The RSI clinic handbook : life beyond the carpal tunnel / Heather Tick.

ISBN 0-9782155-0-8

        1. Overuse injuries--Popular works. 2. Carpal tunnel syndrome—Popular works. I. Title.

RD97.6.T52 2007   617.1'72   C2007-903060-2

Back cover photo by David Amoils Photography
Drawings by Timothy Garrett (timothygarrett.com), Seth Gilbert and Hazel Hewitt
Cover design by James Jigme Glenn

Dedication

This book is dedicated to my parents, Faiga and Samuel Tick.

From my Mother I learned an appreciation for things that were basic, natural and simple. She cooked every meal, from scratch. I also learned about intuition from her. Returning to First Principles has been the foundation of my professional life. My Father taught me about kindness and gentleness and the value of perseverance, hard work and friendship. Because of my heritage, I learned to value time-honored traditions but also to embrace change as an inevitability.

With all my love.

"Prevention is better than treatment, because it saves the labor of being sick."

Dr. Thomas Adams, a 17th century physician

Prologue

In 1993, Mark Gilbert and I started a clinic as a facility that would address the growing epidemic of work related injuries arising in workers who were in sedentary jobs or who did repetitive tasks. There were controversies at that time and even questions about the very existence of RSI and the category to which most of these ailments belonged—myofascial disorders. Dwayne van Eerd joined us at the start and we had other excellent therapists who worked with us in our efforts to provide good quality, effective therapies for a set of conditions that was poorly understood and even more poorly treated by the medical and therapy communities. We ended up calling the facility, The RSI Clinic, because RSI had become the popular name for these conditions even though it was not the most accurate term. As the years passed we developed our ideas and adapted our strategies to be more effective. We learned from the researchers in the field, from innovative therapists and also from the people who had these conditions, what worked and what did not. This book is an attempt to pull together in one place what we have learned and to put it into a concise readable form so people can educate themselves about this group of conditions, their cause and their treatment. Knowledge in this area is a key to prevention of these injuries. It also can help people pursue proper diagnosis and treatment if they have these conditions.

At around the same time as the RSI Clinic came into being, Paul Taylor, the health journalist for the Globe and Mail, wrote a landmark series of articles on Repetitive Strain Injuries. He himself had the condition and he wrote about his experiences with getting a proper diagnosis and treatment. He explored innovative therapies in near and distant places. Paul's integrity as a well-known journalist and his openness about his own condition helped to lend credibility to the existence of RSI. His search for effective therapies helped to focus our own efforts for treatment. Our clinic benefited from his willingness to share his journey in these articles.

There is still a lot of confusion about the names of these injuries and they are often lumped together under the term "Carpal Tunnel Syndrome" (CTS). There is a specific test for CTS that is performed by a variety of specialists. A patient can be seen to either have CTS or not—based on the results of the electrical test, sometimes with complete disregard for the physical findings in closely related structures. The certainty of the test makes some people feel the diagnosis is more legitimate and therefore people (medical and non-medical) have come to regard CTS as a diagnosis "you can hang your hat on". In reality the specific diagnosis of CTS is less important than the bigger picture of the injury. Many patients come to us with the label of CTS, but only a small percentage actually has that specific condition. I have attempted to explain why this confusion has arisen and to point to more useful ways of categorizing RSI.

This phenomenon highlights one of the problems with modern medicine. A century ago medicine placed much more emphasis on the medical history (the story the patient told) and the physical examination. Throughout the 20th century many tests were developed—blood tests, x-rays, CT, MRI, Ultrasound, and nerve conduction tests. These tests give a lot of useful information and have become regarded as "objective" meaning that they do not depend on the opinion of the patient. As the century progressed, the pressure from insurance companies and others encouraged the use of ONLY these "objective" tests in making decisions. Patient history and clinical examination (which is also objective because it does not depend on the opinion of the patient) were considered less important. This left an unfortunate situation: if there was no test for a condition then it was sometimes implied that the condition did not exist or was in the patient's head. For this reason in the

1950's patients with Multiple Sclerosis were sometimes committed to psychiatric facilities because there was no test to explain their bizarre set of problems. In the 1980's, those with RSI were similarly accused of inventing their own problems and a debate raged in the medical community involving authorities who lined up, putting the weight of their hefty reputations on one side or the other. RSI was either seen as a medical condition that had not yet been fully characterized, or it was seen as an excuse for lazy employees.

Our clinic has been a facility, which focused on treating people—we cared for our patients, most of whom found us through word of mouth. We have developed our knowledge by learning from the people affected by these conditions and developed our methods to respond to their needs. The clinic was integrated in its use of practitioners from a wide variety of disciplines. It also had a model of treating each patient as an integrated individual encompassing mind, body and spirit. Research is very important in order to establish mechanisms of injury and healing and to establish best practices. Over the last few years we have become more involved in research and hope to expand this aspect of our work. But we will never lose sight of those who have taught us our most valuable lessons—our patients.

Acknowledgments

No work of this sort is done without a great debt to others. I gratefully acknowledge the clinicians who went before me and from whose methods I learned. They are the early pioneers in this area who withstood the derision of colleagues who disputed the existence of myofascial injuries. I had the privilege of learning from Drs. Janet Travell and Robert Gerwin. Dr. C Chan Gunn has been my mentor over many years since 1991 when I was first introduced to his work through the Acupuncture Foundation of Canada. Every opportunity I have to hear him speak improves my understanding and practice. His teachings synthesized many disparate pieces of information into a coherent theory of myofascial pain that has taken the treatment of such injuries one giant step forward.

I have always had the privilege to work with a wonderful team of therapists and professionals who have shared their knowledge and skills: Mark Gilbert, Dwayne van Eerd, Mark Erwin, Gordon Ko, Lois Singer, Margaret Ranger, Tiziana Schiafone, Scott Whitmore, Angus Driver, Mary Naumovsky, Michelle Katz, Ranil Kumara, John Beverly, David Slater, Andrew Appel, Line Troster, Lisa Beech-Hawley, Fraser McDonald, Linda Finn and Ed Krolow. The researchers at the University of Waterloo, Department of Kinesiology have expanded the understanding of RSI: Howard Green, Donald Ranney, Richard Wells, Jack Callahan and Stu McGill. Linda Rapson, Sona Tahan and Joe Wong of the Acupuncture Foundation of Canada have shared their knowledge generously. Eileen Burford Mason has helped me to get past the limitations of my profession when trying to understand nutrition. I also want to thank Mel Litman for pointing me in an unexpected direction and thereby expanding my knowledge base.

I am extremely grateful to Chandra Teitscheid who has provided me with invaluable advice about the book business and has guided the promotion of this book. I would also like to thank Lisa Dunn and Sharon Foley for their help and patience over the years. Michael Smalley helped me choose a title for this book.

In the editing and organization of this book I gratefully acknowledge the work of Paul Taylor, Aviad Haramati, Mark Gilbert, Seth Gilbert, Emma Tick Gilbert, Noah Gilbert, Dwayne van Eerd and Mark Erwin.

The art work was done by Tim Garrett and Seth Gilbert.

Finally, in their support of all my endeavours, I thank my children Noah, Emma and Seth. My husband Mark has been instrumental in the development of the direction of my career and has supported the production of this book in countless ways. His willingness to think "outside the box" and to follow his heart in our personal and professional lives has been an inspiration.

About the Contributors

Heather Tick MA, MD, CCFP is a Clinical Assistant Professor, University of Arizona, Department of Family and Community Medicine. She is the co-founder and present director of The RSI Clinic and Integrated Pain Treatment Centre in Toronto. She also directs an integrative pain clinic in Tucson Arizona. Dr. Tick has treated thousands of patients with Repetitive Strain Injuries and other myofascial disorders. She is a frequent presenter on the topic of RSI, integrative pain treatment, ergonomics and healthful living. She is currently working on research projects with the department of Kinesiology, University of Waterloo and the University of Arizona.

Mark Gilbert MD, FRCPc, is the co-founder of The RSI Clinic. He is currently the Director of Consultation-Liaison Psychiatry and The Mind-Body Small Group Program at the University of Arizona.

Dwayne van Eerd has degrees in Kinesiology and Health Research Methodology. He is involved in many research projects with the Institute of Work and Health, in Toronto and has presented to many organizations regarding RSI. He continues to have a small clinical practice treating patients with RSI.

Mark Erwin DC, PhD (medical sciences) holds an appointment in the Department of Surgery, division of orthopedics, at the University of Toronto. His clinical work involves the chiropractic treatment of a full range of disorders of the spine. His groundbreaking research is in the field of regenerative medicine, with particular interest in the intervertebral discs of the spine.

Table of Contents

• 1 •
RSI – What is it?

Definition of Repetitive Strain Injuries

"Musculoskeletal symptoms affecting work activities caused by physical and/or psychological stressors on the body, beyond it's ability to adapt."

Sheila is a 32 year old bank employee who was working in a customer service call centre. She was on the phone with customers and was using the computer at the same time. Until 2 years ago she did not have a headset and held the phone between her shoulder and ear by tilting her head to the side. The keyboard was up on a desk and she had to reach up to use it. Sheila sat at her desk all day with only a short break at lunch. She drank coffee and cola through the day.

At first, Sheila noticed soreness in her neck that came and went. It was worse by the end of the workweek and she would feel better after the weekend. She was a "outdoors" type and was active in hiking and sports. About six months later she began to notice that her grip on the tennis racket was not as strong. She began to wake up in the night with pain in her right shoulder and arm. Finally, she began dropping things that were held in her right hand. After a friend wondered if she had Multiple Sclerosis, Sheila got scared and she decided to see the doctor.

What caused Sheila's symptoms?

There are many factors that contribute to the development of the injuries in each individual. Sheila has an injury caused by strained muscles. Some people develop injuries quickly and others can do the same work and remain healthy throughout their career.

Why does this happen?

There are also many theories about what is the underlying cause of muscle strain in repetitive injuries. We don't have all the answers yet.

How can it be prevented?

There are safer work practices that workers and employers can adopt. These can help prevent injuries.

We will explore to these key questions throughout the book.

Repetitive Strain Injuries (RSI) refer to the soft tissue, work relevant disorders that are occurring with increasing frequency in workers doing jobs involving static postures (i.e.: keeping most of the big muscles in the body still) and repetitive motion (i.e.: using the smaller muscle groups for activities like keyboarding, mousing, writing, scanning groceries, grasping tools or manipulating objects etc.) Often workers will present to doctors or other health care providers with localized symptoms which may involve any body part from the neck, shoulders, upper back, and upper limbs extending all the way down to the fingertips. Rarely they will complain of all of the above. Some workers will also develop lower back discomfort and related injuries because of sitting. Low back problems are especially common in industries, which involve repetitive lifting or twisting.

The vast majority of these injuries involve a more extensive area than the presenting symptoms would suggest. A careful examination of the upper limbs, shoulders, upper back and neck often reveals tight bands in the affected muscles, restricted range of motion and tenderness. There may also be weakness, hypersensitivity, poor circulation and puffiness of the overlying skin reported by patients. There is often also very poor posture by the time workers are symptomatic. When so many areas are affected with these injuries, the symptoms can actually move around depending on the activity pattern of the individual. This can be disconcerting to the worker and those providing treatment (not to mention the insurers.)

How do I know I have RSI?

If static postures and/or repetitive activities (work related or not) cause the following:
  + Discomfort, stiffness, numbness or tingling, change in colour or temperature of your shoulders, neck, back, hips or limbs.

- Symptoms that may go away after a brief time of rest but return quickly when you resume the repetitive activity
- The time for the return of the symptoms gets shorter and the time needed to recover gets longer.

If you have these symptoms, see a healthcare professional who is knowledgeable about RSI or myofascial injuries.

The two major movements of the wrist are:

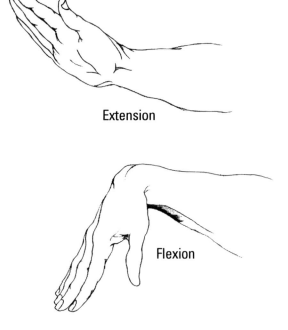

Extension

Flexion

• 2 •
The Magnitude of the Problem

The year is 1654 and Flavio who was educated by the friars is very proud to be able to work as a scribe and help to produce books for the monastery. He carefully dips his quill into the ink and forms the letters on the pages meticulously. There has been talk of a new invention that will make the work easier. The metal pen will hold more ink and not need to be dipped as frequently. The end won't break off like the quills do. That will save time. He hates having to repeatedly clean up the broken end of the quill 10 times an hour. A few of the friars have used the metal pens and Flavio wishes he could use one.

Six months after starting to use a metal pen, Flavio starts to get cramping in his hand. He does not understand why. He is working much faster and can stay with the task of writing for much longer with his new instrument. Why have the cramps begun?

Repetitive strain injuries have been described in the medical literature dating back to the 1700 in *De morbis artificum diatriba* (Diseases of Workers) by Ramazzini. He spoke of hand pain and numbness, and upper limb disability, which developed in scribes due to, repeated movements of their hands in the same direction. There was likely sporadic use of metal pens in ancient times and into the Middle Ages. The widespread replacement of quills due to the manufacturing of the steel nib pen beginning in the 1820's led to an "outbreak" of writers' cramp.

In recent times government and industry are beginning to comprehend the magnitude of these injuries and the advantages of preventative programs. The Occupational Safety and Health Administration of the US Department of Labor (OSHA) estimates that Musculoskeletal Disorders or MSD's (the US term for RSI) affect 1.8 million U.S. workers and account for one third of the most serious on-the-job injuries. They are very costly injuries. US statistics suggest that the direct costs at $15 billion to $20 billion (US$) per year with indirect costs increasing that total to $45 billion to $54 billion (US$). The Industrial Accident Prevention Association, in Canada, cites that between 1996— 2004, RSIs accounted for 42% of all lost time claims, 47% of all lost time claim costs, and 55% of all lost time days among their member companies. Repetitive motion injuries result in more lost workdays than other injuries. It takes longer for workers to recover from carpal tunnel injuries (one type of RSI) than from fractures or amputations.

But the news is not all bad. OSHA has concluded that the key to reducing these costs lies in early reporting and prevention. The OSHA web site reports on one company that reduced workers' compensation costs from $514,000 in 1991 to $176,000 in 1997 by instituting a program of educational seminars. Another company replaced chairs and invested in footrests and adjustable height tables. As a result they reduced compensation costs from $96,000 to $4,500 and at the same time increased employee satisfaction and productivity. OSHA estimates that $1 of every $3 spent on compensation costs is related to improper ergonomics.

In the early 1990's a major North American daily newspaper, like many others, was plagued by RSI. They instituted a program of reorganizing workstations using ergonomics principles, began an educational program for their employees regarding injury prevention and work place stretching, and encouraged and paid for quality care geared for RSI. Within 2 years they had no lost time claims for RSI and they received the maximum possible refund from Workers Compensation.

.

• 3 •
The Injuries
What causes muscle strain?

by Heather Tick and Mark Erwin

Cast of Characters in the Musculoskeletal System

MUSCLES Collections of fibers that can contract—usually in the same direction so that the contraction of a muscle causes a joint to bend or stretch out. Muscles have blood vessels and nerves passing through them to get to other structures. Nerve and blood supplies also are needed for the needs of the muscle itself. Muscles give stability as well as movement.

LIGAMENTS Bands of connective tissue that join bone to bone.

TENDONS Bands of connective tissue that join muscle or other soft tissue to bone.

FASCIA Connective tissue that surrounds and supports muscles, bones and joints.

BONES Hard tissues that support the body and help us move. Bones act as a reservoir of nutrients especially minerals, for use by the rest of the body when needed.

CONNECTIVE TISSUE If you take away all your muscles, bones, internal organs, blood vessels and nerves you would still be left with something that has the form of your body. It would be made of connective tissue. The significance of this "body" is just beginning to be explored. There is fascinating research by Helene Langevin MD, which is exploring the function of what medicine has long regarded as inert filler.

Suzanna is a hairdresser. She has developed a painful right shoulder and her doctor has told her she has bursitis—inflammation of the bursa, which is a small pouch designed to help the tendons of the shoulder slide smoothly over each other. She was given an anti-inflammatory medication and went to see a physiotherapist. She felt some relief for a few weeks. She has kept working and as the weeks go by, she realizes she is getting worse instead of better.

Our bodies were designed to do thousands of different movements each day. The human body ended up in its current configuration after hundreds of thousands of years of evolution that required walking, running, climbing, reaching, lifting and other active movements. It is only in the past 75-100 years that we have moved progressively towards a sedentary lifestyle. People who sit at a desk, work long hours and drive almost everywhere have an increased risk of many diseases, including diabetes and obesity. Therefore it is hardly surprising that people develop symptoms associated with this 'artificial' existence of sedentary lifestyle because it might not 'jive' with the human body that's built to move. People were designed for movement.

Workers with sedentary jobs are doing thousands of repetitions of essentially *similar* movements each day. We need to think of sedentary workers as elite athletes—doing something very remarkable with their bodies. Like all athletes they need to condition and train for the activity and generally take care of their bodies. In the case of repetitive tasks, training involves working in proper postures and with healthy habits. That means, for example, taking frequent short breaks, stretching adequately, recognizing the early signs of injuries to muscles and knowing how to take preventative action. By the time people go to the doctor they are already injured and require treatment, and effective treatment has to address many of these associated factors.

The first time an injured worker presents to the doctor with a complaint she or he may get a diagnosis that focuses on the area that hurts: extensor tendonitis (tennis elbow), flexor tendonitis (golfer's elbow), deQuervains' tenosynovitis, rotator cuff tendonitis, bursitis, etc.—and the cause of the injury, and its connection to the other body parts goes unacknowledged. "Itis" means 'inflammation'. Because many of the labels given to the RSI injuries are "itises," the most common response is to reach for anti-inflammatory drugs— whether prescribed or over the counter. Unfortunately, in chronic injuries, these drugs are of only minimal, symptomatic benefit and they are of no advantage in addressing the underlying causes or to stimulate healing. With early injuries, these drugs can be of help. In many chronic injuries, inflammation is not a major part of the problem and the term "opathy" as in tendonopathy (disorder of the tendon) is a better description. In any case, the larger picture needs to be assessed and addressed. Because of the time constraints and the ways in which doctors and other healthcare professionals have been taught to focus during their schooling, sometimes the tendency is to attend to the area that hurts and not to examine other parts of the body that may be connected.

Let's look at Suzanna's injury. Bursitis, like the one Suzanna has, is one example where chronic inflammation often does play a role in the injury. Inflammation is not always a bad thing—it is the primary method that the body's healing mechanisms are called into play. Inflammation marks the initial steps in a complex series of events that the body needs in order to initiate repair, such as, the migration of white blood cells, increased circulation, the activation of various growth factors, remodeling factors and the like. The downside to inflammation is that it can hurt. The other issue is that unchecked or chronic inflammation is a bad thing. Sometimes the body just isn't able to repair itself and its attempts to do so get stuck in a cycle that continues to wear the body down. A good example is the chronic painful shoulder. Many people may have heard of 'bursitis' in the shoulder. It is very treatable in a variety of ways, however what is paramount and is often missed is why is the bursa inflamed? An example might be Suzanna who cuts hair everyday and develops a painful shoulder. She has gone to her doctor and/or therapist and received therapy that gives some improvement in symptoms. But the problem tends to recur, or, in the worst case scenario, it never gets better. Why? Suzanna performs daily activity with her elbows elevated with her arms parallel to the floor. This position perpetuates the problem and causes her RSI. So, in addition to therapy, the biomechanics of the problem must be considered. Suzanna can keep cutting hair, but needs to lower her elbows to her side. She may need to stand on a box to achieve this. This will change the angle of the arms and will decrease the constant pinching of the shoulder muscles, tendons and bursa. When only the inflammation part of the bursitis is treated the tissues can't repair themselves. An assessment of Suzanna's neck alignment may reveal that she often holds her head

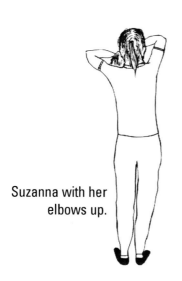

Suzanna with her
elbows up.

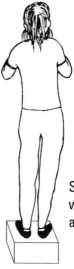

Suzanna on a box
with her elbows
at her side.

in a tilted position for hours on end and has developed tight muscles at the sides of her neck. These tight muscles squeeze the nerves as they exit from the spinal cord at the side of the neck on their way down to the shoulders and upper limbs. If her neck muscles are treated then the nerves are no longer squeezed and the shoulder tissues can heal more quickly. In this case posture, myofascial injuries and inflammation are all part of Suzanna's problem.

There are long and short term consequences of poor posture. Sitting often leads to posture with the chin and shoulders slouched forward. In the short term there may be muscle pain in the neck and shoulders. However, the long-term implications for the neck are much more serious. The oral surgeons tell us that every inch that the head is held forward of its neutral position doubles the effective load on the neck (See the bowling ball pictures in Chapter 5). The discs, bones, joints and ligaments adapt to load by changing shape over time. Constant and excessive abnormal load have been proven to be related to the development of disc problems. Therefore bad posture speeds up the development of degenerative disc disease. Sitting, even with good posture, imposes a 5 fold

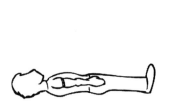
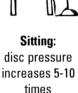
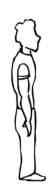

Sitting:
disc pressure
increases 5-10
times

Standing:
disc pressure
increases 3-5
times

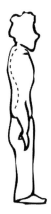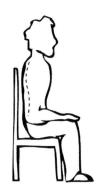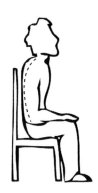

increase in pressure within the discs of the low back as compared to the pressures encountered with lying down. Standing imposes a 3-5 fold increase in disc pressure. Slouching in a chair increases the load on the discs up to 10 fold. This is one of the reasons why people with disc problems feel much better walking than sitting or standing in one place. Certainly the position of the spine while sitting is very important insofar as the progression of disc disease is concerned. Maintaining the normal, neutral curves of the spine while sitting is imperative because the 'slouched' position that commonly occurs results in a 'C' shaped, rather than the normal 'S' shaped spine. Prolonged sitting has been reported to cause cumulative, irreversible damage to the discs of the spine-with predictable consequences: pain, muscle spasm and and wearing down of the discs and vertebrae. Sometimes adjusting one's low back posture will improve the problem of upper back and neck pain in workers doing prolonged deskwork.

Whether it is pain in the wrist, elbow, forearm, shoulder, hips or back that is the initial symptom, many of the underlying problems may be the same—posture, poor biomechanical positions, repetitive motion and some inflammation. It is therefore important to assess people comprehensively even when they seem to have a very focused complaint, like wrist or elbow pain. There is a need to assess and correct posture, muscle tightness, muscle compensation patterns, muscle imbalances and weakness.

> The presenting symptom is only the tip of the iceberg.

• 4 •
A rose by any other name...

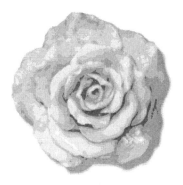

"Good doctors use both individual clinical expertise and the best available external evidence, and neither alone is enough. Without clinical expertise, practice risks becoming tyrannized by evidence, for even excellent external evidence may be inapplicable to or inappropriate for an individual patient. Without current best evidence, practice risks becoming rapidly out of date, to the detriment of patients."

DL Sackett, WMC Rosenberg, JA Muir Gray, RB Haynes, WS Richardson

Fred is an accountant who came into the office and started by saying he was confused, his employer was confused and his insurance company was asking questions that neither one could answer.

After working on a particularly difficult case of a company that was being audited, Fred's right hand started to go painful and numb. He had put in a great deal of overtime lately, and the client was really stressed throughout the process. Fred went to his family doctor to find out what was wrong. The family doctor examined Fred's wrist and said she thought it might be Carpal Tunnel syndrome (a condition where a nerve in the wrist is squeezed). The doctor gave him an anti-inflammatory and sent him to see a physiotherapist (PT).

The PT examined Fred's hand and elbow and the muscles of the forearm (the part of the upper limb between the wrist and elbow). The PT said Fred might have carpal tunnel, but he was more concerned with the tendonitis at the elbow—the inflamed, tender tendons. The PT initiated treatment of the elbow with some therapy for the wrist as well.

Fred did not notice much improvement and after 3 weeks he went to see the chiropractor that his friend sees. The chiropractor examined his neck and said there were bones out of place and that manipulation would help. Fred started regular manipulation and was given exercises for home. He found the treatments lasted a very short while and after 3 weeks he was still in a lot of pain with a little improvement in the numbness.

He filed to go off on short term disability. He needed notes from his treating professionals. The forms filled out for the insurance company from the doctor, PT and chiropractor each contained a different diagnosis—carpal tunnel, tendonitis, neck strain. Fred came into my office and said both he and the insurance company wanted to know which one was the correct diagnosis.

After a thorough examination of the musculoskeletal system including the neck, mid back, low back, hips, shoulders, upper arms, forearms, elbows, wrists and hands, I told Fred that they were all correct diagnoses. And what is more there were more diagnostic names to add to the list.

The names we give to things are very important because they can change how we think of them. This is especially important in medicine. When the names we use are accurate they can help communicate information; when inaccurate, they can confuse what we assume about the condition and what we may reach for as a treatment. This chapter will discuss the names that are applied to muscular injuries from two different perspectives—firstly, looking at specific injuries and secondly, more generally relating to larger diagnostic categories that sometimes get confused with each other.

PART 1

As was discussed in Chapter 3, when the injury that a person has is called an "itis," (such as tendonitis), which in medical terminology means "inflammation," this name suggests that the proper treatment for this condition includes ice and anti-inflammatories. In some acute cases this approach is useful but in most chronic cases there is little "itis" or inflammation and the name obscures the true nature of the problem.

In medicine, the purpose of nomenclature (naming) is to convey information in an accurate way, which helps to describe the condition and draw links with other similar conditions. Sometimes it is useful to be as specific as possible: when a bone is broken it is useful to know exactly which part of what bone is affected. With chronic muscle and soft tissue problems (such as whiplash, rotator cuff injuries, most cases of carpal tunnel and thoracic outlet syndrome, de Quervains' tenosynovitis, extensor and flexor tendonitis, lumbar strain, piriformis syndrome and post surgical failed back) it would be clearer to use more general terms because many of these conditions exist together most of the time. If we take one step back from the specific labels above we could use terms like tension neck or shoulder hand syndrome. We can become even more generalized with such terms as myofascial pain syndrome (*myo* means muscle and *fascia* supports and connects the muscles and other structures). This latter term describes the pathophysiology— what is wrong and with what structure. It also acknowledges that the structures are connected and they don't work in isolation in the body. As the song goes "the thigh bone's connected to the hip bone." It is similar to using a wide-angle lens rather than a microscope. You get a very different perspective of the scene with the wide-angle lens; patterns and relationships may be clearer.

In certain circles, though, the microscope is very popular—insurers want to be as specific as they can be in order to limit liability; surgeons need to be focused by the very nature of the intervention they make. And so there is pressure to keep using a microscope. The insurers certainly have a dilemma. It is best described by "claim creep", the term used to describe how an individual gets entitlement for an insurance claim for a certain body part and then progressively tries to add on the adjacent body parts to extend the claim. The insurers have a legitimate concern. The claimant has an equally difficult position because the right shoulder that may be the recognized injury, really is connected to the right arm and forearm and even the left shoulder. All those other structures may get overused as the result of the original area of complaint. Naming these conditions for the one body part that is most symptomatic sometimes prevents people from looking at the whole. Someone with carpal tunnel syndrome needs to have not only their hand and wrist examined, but also their forearm (for tight extensors and especially flexors), arm (for tight biceps), shoulder for problems with the rotator cuff muscles that can interfere with shoulder movement, neck (for decreased range of motion) and even their back (for compensatory patterns because their neck is a mess). A careful examination will often reveal problems in these other areas. It is therefore more helpful to call the condition MFPS (Myofascial Pain Syndrome) and specify the areas affected, such as, "MFPS in the distribution of the cervical spine (neck) on the left affecting primarily rotator cuff, scalenes and forearm."[1]

PART 2

MFPS, FM, CFS, RSD, CRPS—Painfully Confusing

There is a lot of confusion concerning the above conditions because some are poorly understood and because there is a lot of overlap of symptoms among them. Laboratory tests are also not helpful for the most part in making these diagnoses.

MFPS stands for Myofascial Pain Syndrome. It has a clear cause, a clear pattern in its presentation (if you know what to look for) and series of treatments that can be helpful in its treatment. The presence of trigger points (tight tender bands in the muscles) is the hallmark of MFPS. Most RSI from repetitive activities is myofascial in nature.

We tend to look at the musculoskeletal system as static rather than involved in a constant dynamic process of injury and healing. In fact, there is a constant breakdown and rebuilding of the cells in our body. It has been estimated that every 2 years we make enough cells for a whole new person.

All the body tissues, including muscles, are involved in an extensive program for the maintenance of their own health. There are continuous small injuries and ongoing efforts of the muscles to

---

[1] A recent review article in the Journal of Clinical Epidemiology, suggests a change to a more general and inclusive system of naming, (Van Eerd et al) such as MSD or musculoskeletal disorder. Van Eerd D et al **Classification for upper-limb musculoskeletal disorders in workers: a review of the literature.** J Clin Epidemiol 2003.

One of the most helpful descriptions of myofascial disorders is an analogy that is used by Dr C. Chan Gunn in his book "The Gunn Approach to the Treatment of Chronic Pain: Intramuscular Stimulation for Myofascial Pain of Radiculopathic Origin."

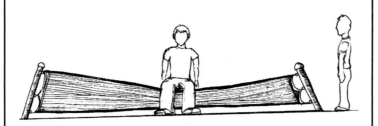

There is someone who is sitting on a tennis net and causing the posts to lean towards the middle. Most of the helping professions are focused on the posts (the bones) where the symptom is. They may x-ray them, try to push them back, reinforce the posts, and transplant them to put them closer to the middle. But none of these interventions will have any lasting effect, because there is someone sitting on the tennis net. The net is the muscle and it is shortened because of the net-sitter. Getting the sitter off the net will allow a definitive intervention to correct the posts. Then, Dr. Gunn points out, there is still the boss of the net-sitter over in the corner—that is the nerve that governs the function of the muscle. So after the muscle is lengthened by a local intervention, the health of the nerve also needs to be improved with specific treatment.

(used with the permission of Professor C. Chan Gunn)

heal themselves. When we see an injury that does not heal, it is because the balance between injury and healing has been tipped and the healing can't keep up. When muscles are damaged, the injured areas shorten into tight bands often called trigger points. The shortened muscles then cause pulling where the muscles attach (to tendon, bone or other structures), interfere with blood flow and cause subtle pressure on nerves. These secondary problems often are the cause of the symptoms, which bring patients in for treatment. But it is important to follow the symptoms back to their root cause—the tightened muscles.

FM or Fibromyalgia is a complex condition, which as yet has no clear set of causes or treatments. Often those with pain that has lasted a long time will receive a diagnosis of FM even though they do not meet the criteria set out for the diagnosis.

The National Fibromyalgia Association website defines FM as:

[1] Widespread pain in all four quadrants of the body for a minimum duration of three months

[2] Tenderness or pain in at least 11 of the 18 specified tender points when pressure is applied

---

It is usually associated with a sleep disorder. The early literature suggested that people not be given the label of FM if they have another diagnosis that can explain chronic pain and ill health. These criteria for FM are used to give some consistency to the study of FM but they do not reflect a cause or influence the decisions about treatment. This is a confusing area for people with FM and those who diagnose and treat them. FM and MFPS are often confused because the initials are the reverse of each other, both conditions have points on the body that are tender (FM has tender points and MFPS has trigger points which are **not** the same thing).

CFS or Chronic Fatigue Syndrome is the subject of a lot a fascinating research. There is mounting evidence that CFS and FM are conditions in which there are abnormalities in the energy producing mechanisms in muscle. There is likely overlap between these conditions. Research is indicating that CFS is a disorder of the immune system that causes a myositis (inflammation of muscles), a decrease in some aspects of heart function and other symptoms based on immune dysfunction. Recent studies are pointing to a genetic susceptibility and an environmental factors coming together to produce the syndrome. They are currently working on a new name for CFS.

Some people with FM also have MFPS and it is sometimes difficult to tell which symptoms come from which condition. It's like trying to sort out which apple made a particular part of the applesauce.

RSD, or Reflex Sympathetic Dystrophy, has been given a new name—Chronic Regional Pain Syndrome or CRPS. CRPS can be associated with chronic pain. The field of chronic pain is very confusing. There has been a tremendous amount of very interesting research but we are still at the stage of having 75 pieces out of a 5000 piece jigsaw puzzle. In some individuals it is still difficult to understand what causes their pain and what interferes with achieving pain relief. It seems that in chronic pain the sympathetic nervous system gets unbalanced to variable degrees. (There is the somatic nervous system under voluntary control and the autonomic nervous system, which is divided into the sympathetic and parasympathetic nervous system, which balance each other. The sympathetic system is for fight-or-flight reactions.)

In some cases of RSD or CRPS there are unmistakable signs of the unbalanced sympathetic system—coldness of a limb, excess sweating, colour changes to the skin and sometimes changes to the texture of the skin called dystrophic changes and stiffness of movement. The extreme cases are unmistakable. Many people have more subtle signs that can be missed, or are just brought out under certain conditions. In MFPS there are subtle signs of sympathetic dysfunction that are caused by the compression of nerves by tight muscles.

Summary

Ideally a naming system should help to clarify and delineate similarities and differences. But we have not yet reached that point with these conditions. Research has greatly advanced our understanding , but there is much more work to be done. One of the reasons for the controversy about RSI has been the lack of adequate research to explain how and why these disorders develop in some people. In general chronic conditions are harder to study than acute ones. Research being conducted by Dr. Howard Green and his team at the University of Waterloo is finding disturbances with energy production mechanisms in the affected muscles of those with longstanding cases of RSI. This suggests a legitimate biological source of the disorder. Other recent studies have identified a class of immune cells called microglia, which wrap themselves around the axons (long segments of nerve cells that carry messages) and secrete a substance in people with chronic pain. As we develop a greater understanding of the mechanisms of these conditions, perhaps there will be a more logical naming system as well as more treatments available to reverse the process and speed up healing.

But it is useful to remember that the world does not define itself according to scientific principles. The theory of relativity was a more thorough explanation of the universe even when Newtonian physics was all we had. We just didn't know it. So science is always striving to catch up to reality—not the other way around. We need to search for the evidence and remember that just because something needs further research does not mean that it is without merit. Physicians used to prescribe x-rays for acne. As people developed thyroid cancers from the radiation this form of treatment was abandoned. In the 1970's and 80's the medical establishment laughed at the notion that infection played a role in stomach ulcers. In 2005 the Nobel Prize was awarded to Drs. Marshall and Warren for their discovery of H. Pylori, the bacterium that causes ulcers. We would do well to have humility in the face of the phenomenal complexity of human physiology. Some of today's certainties will soon be on the shelf along with yesterday's snake oil. We need to strive for evidence to support our proposed treatments and it is always best to approach these issues with an open mind and a close collaboration between physician and patient. The labels we use are of secondary importance.

There is an increasing awareness of the need for medicine to reintegrate its parts into a more holistic approach to patients because they are more than a collection of distinct parts. The term being used to signal this approach is Integrative Medicine. It

---

The Consortium of Academic Health Centers for Integrative Medicine, **(an organization dedicated to medical education and research) has the following definition of Integrative Medicine:**

Integrative Medicine is the practice of medicine that reaffirms the importance of the relationship between practitioner and patient, focuses on the whole person, is informed by evidence, and makes use of all appropriate therapeutic approaches, healthcare professionals and disciplines to achieve optimal health and healing.

---

involves integration of care of the individual as well as cooperation with and integration of other healing disciplines.

The original 8 Institutions who formed the consortium are as follows: Duke University, Harvard University, Stanford University, University of California, San Francisco, University of Arizona, University of Maryland, University of Massachusetts, and the University of Minnesota. There are currently 32 esteemed University members.

• 5 •
Common Presentations

Let's return to Fred's first appointment at the clinic.

He fills out an extensive intake form which asks about his symptoms, how they started and many associated features. He also has to record his past medical and surgical history, his medication history, his eating, smoking and drinking habits. He is asked about supplements and over the counter medications as well as past treatments. He fills out a pain diagram as well.

Fred is then seen by the intake physician who reviews all this information with him and asks more detailed questions about the present condition and any items from his history that may be associated. The doctor asks in more detail about Fred's work habits. Any unresolved general medical issues are discussed to assess their relevance to Fred's current problems. A family history is taken to see if there are any hereditary or environmental factors which need attention and also to get some preliminary information on Fred's social support network.

The physical examination involves an examination of Fred's neck and back, a review of how he moves from his feet to his shoulders, arms and hands. Subtle signs of muscle dysfunction, arthritis are noted.

Fred asks the doctor why she examined his low back and asked about his family history when he has a work related arm disability. She explains that she sees the body as an integrated whole and though the back may not be the source of the injury, the way he sits affects his neck and therefore the nerve supply to his arms.

The physician then tells Fred what the findings are, explains tests that need to be ordered, discusses nutrition, lifestyle changes, supplements if needed, natural remedies that may help and drugs if needed. Proposed therapies are explained. Fred may make another appointment to discuss these issues again, since there has been a lot of information shared in this appointment and he may have questions once he thinks about it all.

Fred leaves, realizing that this is the most thorough assessment and explanation he has had regarding this injury. He starts to see of the connections between his injury and his work habits, his poor diet and his lack of healing. Even though he knows he has to make some changes and take responsibility for his health, he is optimistic that there is hope for improvement.

Regardless of what is the initial presenting symptom of RSI, it is important to thoroughly assess the patient. At the RSI Clinic we have evaluated and treated thousands of people with these injuries and the following reflects the most common patterns of injuries which we see in the group who have upper limb RSI. The way in which Repetitive Strain Injuries (RSI) become a chronic problem has yet to be fully understood. People come to the RSI Clinic with a variety of different symptoms, such as: pain in the wrist, tenderness on either side of the elbow, swelling and discomfort with thumb movements, aching in the neck, shoulders and upper arms. There are many different symptoms but when we examine people with RSI, we see consistent patterns of physical findings that workers have in common.

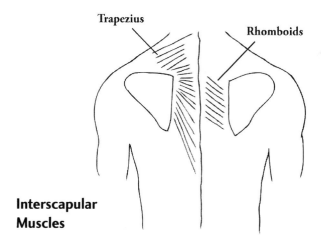

Trapezius

Rhomboids

Interscapular Muscles

One of the first problems is that the muscles between the shoulder blades (the interscapular muscles) stop working properly. (This may happen in computer users, musicians, assembly line workers and anyone with repetitive tasks of the upper limbs and the tendency for poor posture.) The usual work of the interscapular muscles is to help stabilize the shoulder blades so that the upper limbs can perform precise movements. Workers develop poor posture, hunching over their work. The strong pectoral muscles in the front of the chest get tightened and further pull the shoulders forward. This causes the interscapular muscles to become weak. The interscapular muscles therefore must keep working to hold the shoulder blades steady. This is known as a static posture where muscles have to work even though they do not move a body part. These muscles are often the first to get fatigued and then they can't do their job effectively. The rotator cuff muscles (of the shoulder) and some of the neck muscles may then become overworked trying to take over the job of trying to stabilize the shoulder blades. At the same time, the muscles which are activated when the shoulders are hiked upwards—the levator scapulae and the upper fibers of trapezius—can get overworked with static postures and repetitive work (especially when the arms are in the wrong position and under conditions of stress—physical and emotional.)

Seated workers often get into bad habits with the posture of their head and they develop a "chin forward" posture. This can happen for a variety of reasons, such as fatigue causing the head to hang forward, intense concentration, visual demands or problems causing the person to lean towards their work. The head should be aligned over the bony support of the spine and not hung forward. Imagine 2 scenarios:

1) You are holding an 11 to 12 pound bowling ball in your hand and you have it in line with your elbow. This position keeps the ball in line with the support by the bones of the forearm.

2) You are holding the bowling ball with your hand out in front of your elbow.

It's easy to imagine in this case that you can sustain that weight for longer if the ball is over your elbow. Similarly it is easier to hold up your head if you have good posture. With the chin forward posture the muscles of the neck become tightened so that proper posture no longer feels natural. The neck muscles are then constantly overworking and become sore. (See information in Chapter 3 regarding chin forward posture.)

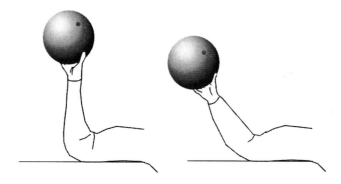

Symptoms in the forearms are more variable and they may depend on the specific tasks of the worker. The **extensor** muscles (the outside of the elbow), the **flexors** (the inside of the elbow) or the **deQuervains'** muscles (the side of the thumb) may be most affected and have tight, tender bands and swelling. There may be pressure on the median nerve as it passes through its entire course beginning as nerve roots in the neck, then as part of the brachial plexus in the arm and forearm. (Nerves that go to the arms begin exit the spine as nerve roots at the level of the neck and then form branches.) If there is additional pressure at the wrist it may be called **Carpal Tunnel Syndrome**. The carpal tunnel is a 1/2 inch long compartment at the wrist where the one vein, artery, and nerve that supply part of the hand pass.

Nodules and pouches of fluid may develop along the tendons of the wrists and hands. Nodules are usually thickened connective tissue and are most common on the palm side of the hand and can prevent the tendons from gliding smoothly. Nodules are associated with "**trigger finger**" when the nodule causes the finger to get stuck when the worker tries to straighten the digit. With further force to straighten the finger there is a snapping sensation when it actually does straighten. **Ganglion cysts** are fluid filled pouches on tendons and are more common on the back of the wrist or hand and can also happen on the palm side. Both of these conditions have traditionally been treated with injections of steroid, and sometimes surgery. Trigger fingers and gangion cysts are both associated with myofascial trigger points and shortening of the muscles of the forearm. They often improve and even disappear with proper myofascial treatments.

Some workers develop **thoracic outlet symptoms (TOS)**—the thoracic outlet is the space at the base of the neck extending towards the axilla (armpit) where major vein, artery and nerve trunks pass from the neck and chest down to the arms. The symptoms of thoracic outlet syndrome (TOS) are pain, weakness, and abnormal sensation due to pressure on the neurovascular bundle (the vein, artery and nerve trunks). Tight scalene muscles (muscles at the base of the neck at the sides) are often a factor for the TOS patients we see.

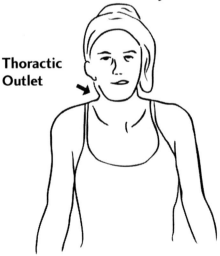

Thoractic Outlet

Carpal Tunnel Syndrome (CTS)

CTS deserves a paragraph of its own because the term is overused and the condition is overdiagnosed to the point that the actual term loses its true meaning. A diagnosis of CTS tends to lead straight to a surgical consultation when in fact the majority of cases do very well with conservative, non surgical treatment. Susan MacKinnon, a well know hand surgeon came to this conclusion in the mid 1990's. Our clinic has been successfully treating CTS with non surgical therapies since we began. As explained in the prologue, a lot of the musculoskeletal disorders or MSDs attract the label of CTS, while only a few people actually have it. For those who do have CTS, it is useful to try conservative treatments before considering surgery. It is helpful to work with a therapist to release the tight muscles that usually are present in the neck, shoulders, upper arms and forearms. Laser therapy may also help to reduce the swelling of tissues around the wrist and relieve pressure on the median nerve at the wrist.

Focal Dystonia

Focal Dystonia can be very distressing because it is uncommon, not completely understood and presents with troubling symptoms. The affected part, often in the hand or fingers, won't listen to the commands. Usually workers will complain that they can't properly control the movement of one of their fingers after they have been doing a repetitive activity for a while. It has been diagnosed in dentists and musicians but can occur with any repetitive work. Likely the muscles or the nerves responsible for the coordination of the movement get fatigued or stuck, like an old fashioned "broken record" playing the same bit of music over and over. We have found that treating the trigger points helps to improve the control over the muscle coordination. Changing the way the worker performs the task is also helpful because that strategy initiates a new motor pattern (like playing a different part of the record.)

Summary

There appears to be a cascade effect in the development of symptoms beginning with the overuse of the interscapular (between the shoulder blades) muscles. Other muscles attempt to compensate but they are not meant to perform the jobs they are asked to do. They quickly become fatigued and begin to cause pain. It is akin to asking your 90-year-old grandmother to go out and shovel the snow because you got tired of doing it.

The feature that all of the above conditions have in common is tightened muscles. It is very important to remember that even though there are different symptoms, the root cause is the same.

> With RSI the symptoms are more variable than the physical evidence—
>
> We see similar physical signs in workers with different jobs and different complaints.

• 6 •
Ergonomics is a Verb
Advice for employers

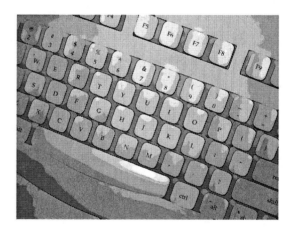

This chapter uses the example of office eronomics: the principles apply to other types of work such as factories and production lines, as well.

These days the term "ergonomic" is used to sell everything from desks to computer mice. The prevailing attitude is that if it says "ergonomic" that it is somehow better and it will prevent the injuries. The merchandisers are pushing a misconception: the idea that the right furniture or accessories will prevent or treat these injuries. The truth of the matter is that Ergonomics is the **act** of fitting the workstation to the individual. Ergonomics is not the furnishings, it is more properly, the activity. It is critical to understand that the most ergonomically designed workstation, *if used improperly*, will not prevent injury.

Ergonomics will not substitute for the treatment of established RSI injuries. However proper ergonomic set up used by educated workers will help prevent injury, reduce disability costs and increase productivity.

Let's take keyboards, for example. There are different sizes and some different configurations (no numeric pad, keys farther apart, QWERTY, DVORAK) and different shapes (curved, split, waterfall). Due to the different sizes of hands, variability in the range of motion at the elbow and wrist, and different keying requirements, one size does not fit all. Therefore, the conscientious employer who wants to prevent injury and so replaces everyone's keyboard with one that is marketed as being "ergonomic" may be adequately serving the needs of only a few of the employees. In the long run, it is more beneficial to have each worker evaluated in their workstation by a knowledgeable assessor and replace only what is really necessary.

Assessment

For small business the words "ergonomics assessment" may seem intimidating (*Sends a shudder through the accounting department*). There may be the fear that the process is too involved, too expensive and commits the employer to an ongoing course of action that they can't control. However, ergonomic improvements can be made in a practical, stepwise fashion that can fit the budgets of small business. The key is to try to utilize the existing set-up and modify it where possible to improve the position of the worker. Suggestions for new equipment can be implemented, as the budget becomes available. The assessment should provide a sense of the order of priorities, as well. That way the company knows how to wisely spend its ergonomics dollars.

Adjustment, Replacement when necessary

A proper ergonomics assessment needs to involve watching the worker in the workstation, looking for work patterns, postures and positions. Often it is possible to alter existing equipment to achieve optimal positioning without buying new equipment. Sometimes only inexpensive accessories such as monitor risers or mouse trays are required. Other times, more extensive purchases are needed to achieve a safe work environment.

Body position is the key to a safe and efficient workplace. For example shoulder muscles are most relaxed when the arms hang naturally by your side. Raising the forearms by bending at the elbow to about 90° is the best keyboard/mouse position (for most people). This position causes less exertion and fatigue in the muscles of the shoulders and between the shoulder blades. The chair arms, keyboard, and mouse platform need to be adjusted to leave the arms in this position. If the existing equipment can't be configured in this way, then it is time to look at new items, which can be properly adjusted.

These days there are some new and exciting developments in the equipment department. Research has shown that the seated posture is very damaging to the discs between the vertebrae of the lumbar spine or lower back.[2] The use of "Sit-Stand" the workstation can be very helpful solution. This means the workstation can be changed from one where the worker sits, to a station where the worker can stand. This used to require great expense and heavy hydraulics. Now there are articulating keyboard trays that will flip up on top of the desk and monitor supports that easily bring the monitor up to an appropriate height as well. So now an option that used to cost thousands of dollars can be offered for hundreds instead. There are now also many shapes and sizes of computer tables, at reasonable cost, which will rise to standing height.

Education

Education is a key component in the prevention and the treatment of workplace injuries. Employees need to be educated regarding the prevention of injuries—good posture during work, rest and stretch breaks, knowledge of how to adjust the furniture and tools at their work stations, the potential impact of non-work activities on the development of injuries, and the benefits of healthy lifestyle for injury prevention. There are many tools for education that we have found beneficial in large and small companies. Lunch and Learn Seminars on safe work habits, good nutritional practices, workplace stretches and recognition of early injuries can help to modify the workplace culture. Handouts or intranet postings for all workers to orient them to safe work habits, stretch techniques and equipment setup can provide on-going sources of information. Our experience has shown us that reinforcing safe work habits and reminders to stretch are important.

---

[2] An interesting book that outlines the physical consequences of sitting is *The Seated Man, Homo Sedens*, by A.C. Mandal (1985). He promotes the use of slanted seats and desk tops so the hips are sloped downwards at greater than a 90° angle and the head does not need to bend forward

Recognizing injuries early often prevents them from progressing further. It also allows the educational material to be reinforced to an individual who may now be more motivated to incorporate it into the daily routine. The cost of treating an early injury is significantly lower and time off work can usually be avoided. It is always preferable to keep people at work. Implementing an "early warning system" requires ongoing dialogue with workers.

Once the workstation is set up properly it is necessary to remember that the way in which the equipment is used is as important as the configuration of the furnishings. Therefore, the key to a safe working environment is education. It is essential to learn proper work techniques, how to adjust the various components of the workstation and how to stretch the neck and forearm muscles effectively. Research has shown that taking stretch breaks not only reduces injuries, but also improves productivity!

Summary

Each year companies spend large amounts of money on new furnishings and equipment. Only sometimes are there adequate considerations given to the people who will use them. The pace and priorities of work in our society has more often been defined by the capacity of the machines and equipment and less often by the capacity of the people. It is important to make sure the company's prevention dollars are spent wisely. Implementing ergonomic changes requires coordinating the equipment changes/adjustments with adequate education.

Overuse syndromes account for an increasingly large percentage of workers' compensation costs each year. The U.S. Bureau of Labor Statistics (BLS) annual survey reports that these injuries represent nearly half of the occupational illnesses reported. Although the statistics are less available, the situation in Canada is likely the same. We are finally beyond the stage of arguing over the existence of these conditions and are now at the point of being able to make meaningful interventions to prevent them, recognize them early and take appropriate action. A proactive approach focusing on education, early recognition, and implementation has been shown to help reduce the numbers and severity of injuries and therefore lower costs to the employer.

When doing workplace ergonomics assessments, I am often astounded that people take so little time to learn how to adjust their equipment. They seem to be so focused on getting on with their work that they do not take the time to look after their own comfort in the workstation. When I show them the proper adjustments, they are often surprised at how comfortable they are. I have seen workers attitudes change after being shown that they have equipment that adjusts to fit THEM. They see the employer as more caring and they have told me they even like the job better!

• 7 •

Office Ergonomics

What to do if you are a worker

by Heather Tick and Dwayne van Eerd

Disclaimer: *Consult your doctor, physical therapist or chiropractor regarding a safe exercise program for you. This is especially important if you are injured or have any medical conditions.*

Muscle Basics:

When muscles are used for repetitive tasks, it is important to do some preventative maintenance in order to avoid injury. The following is a guideline on how to set up your work environment safely.

What are ergonomics?

Ergonomics: "fitting the job to the worker."
In an office environment this can often be accomplished by using adjustable equipment and allowing time for breaks.

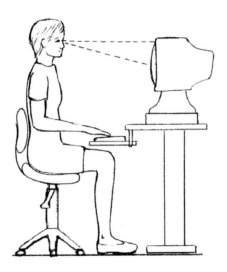

Understand your equipment:

Take the time to understand how to adjust the equipment at your workstation. Each person is different and may therefore require different settings in order to be comfortable. You may re-adjust the equipment throughout your workday to put your body in a slightly different position since this may vary the muscle use patterns.

Remember: Correct equipment if used incorrectly may still lead to injury.

If you have pain that is persistent or severe enough to change the way you work, be sure to see a health professional. Once you have pain it is unlikely that ergonomic changes alone will be enough to correct the problem.

Recommendations for seated posture at the workstation.

Eyes: Facing forward relaxed (i.e. not squinting etc.) Adjust the monitor so that your eyes, when looking straight forward, are viewing the top of the screen.

Neck: In an upright, neutral position allowing your head to be facing forward. Don't lean into the monitor.

Shoulders: Square to the keyboard and monitor and completely relaxed. Don't hunch!

Elbows: Should be close to the body, and bent at approximately or greater than 90°, allowing your arms to hang from your shoulders in a natural position. Forearms should be parallel to the floor or slanted slightly downwards.

Wrists: In a relaxed straight position. Keeping your wrists slightly lower than your elbows usually makes keeping this position easier.

Low back: Supported with the appropriate part of the chair. Usually there is a curved portion of the seat back, which if positioned properly will support your low back with a natural curve.

Knees/Hips: Bent at approximately 90° so that your thighs are approximately parallel to the floor. Be sure to leave three to four fingers of space between the back of your knees and the edge of the chair. Your hips may be slightly higher than your knees.

Feet: Flat on the floor. If your feet can't reach the floor you may need to use a footrest. Only use a footrest if necessary.

Remember these are recommendations that may not be right for everyone. You may need to consult an expert.

Recommendations for the adjustments of workstation components.

It is **NOT** necessary to have adjustable equipment if you can maintain the positions in the following description, with what you have. If more than one person is using a workstation it is usually advisable to have some adjustability in the workstation. Sometimes an adjustable chair is all that is required to make a workstation safe. These are general recommendation and there is controversy in the research about exact specifications. In general, it is helpful to know how to adjust your furniture to get yourself comfortable. Changing things around periodically can also help.

Chair: Adjust the height of the chair to allow you to sit with your feet flat on the floor and your thighs roughly parallel to the floor. Adjust the seatpan so that you can fit four fingers between the back of the knee before the chair seat begins and so that the fullest part of the curve rests in the small of your back (the part of your back that curves inward). If you choose to use armrests make sure they are at the level of your elbow and your shoulders are completely relaxed. If you do use them, do not allow them to interfere with your movements or arm position. Armrests are often useful to support the forearm when mousing.

Kneeling chairs

These chairs enjoyed a brief flurry of popularity. Most people don't find them a good long term solution. However there are some who really like them and find they help with low back problems. Sometimes people complain that the pressure on their knees is unpleasant.

The chair is a key component to workstation comfort. People sit differently. The chair manufacturer, Keilhauer, noticed this principle and a recent study by the University of Waterloo kinesiology department has confirmed that more women prefer to sit forward in front of their sit-bones and a higher percentage of men like to sit behind their sit bones.[3] Make sure the chair accommodates you comfortably in the ways that you like to sit. If the chair back gives you support between the shoulder blades it may help to discourage rounding the shoulders forward into a slouched position. (The sit bones are part of the pelvic bones and they are at the base of you buttocks, close to the seat when you sit.)

---

[3] Clinical Biomechanics, Vol 20, Issue 10,Dec 2005, pp 1101 - 1110. Dunk and Callahan. Dr. Tick was a consultant on this project.

Keyboard tray: Adjust the keyboard tray so that it is at the level of your elbow or slightly below. Bend your elbow to slightly greater than 90° to place your hands in a relaxed position on the keyboard with your wrists in a neutral position (not bent up towards you). Your elbows should hang at your side. Adjust the keyboard and tray (if possible) to allow the keyboard to lay as flat as possible or with a negative tilt (i.e. with the back lower than the front). This will help to achieve a neutral wrist position while typing. If you cannot adjust the keyboard height, then adjust your chair for the best wrist/hand position possible.

If your feet cannot rest flat on the floor once you have your upper body positioned correctly, then use a footrest to support your feet.

> If you have an adjustable height table or a table that is the right height for proper arm position, you may not need a keyboard tray at all.

Mouse: The mouse should be at the same height as the keyboard and placed directly beside the keyboard. It can sometimes be placed on a small tray over the number pad on the right side of the keyboard, if you do not use the number pad often. Minimize the amount of reaching you need to do to use the mouse. Alternate right and left hands if you use the mouse a lot. (Be sure to program the mouse properly for left hand use). If nothing else works put the mouse in front of the keyboard or on a binder in your lap. There are newer mouse and other pointing devices that are incorporated into a wrist rest at the front of the keyboard.

Monitor height: Place the monitor directly in front of you. Adjust it so that your eyes, at level gaze, are at the top of the screen. The monitor should be tilted **slightly** up towards your face. (Avoid too much tilt, as this can result in glare). The screen should be approximately "arm's length" away from you (usually 45 to 60 centimeters away). However adjust this distance so that it is a comfortable reading distance for you. If you wear glasses, or bifocals, you may have to set the monitor closer (and possibly lower) to accommodate your focal length. If you have difficulty finding the optimal distance please check with your ophthalmologist or optometrist. Sometimes special computer glasses are helpful. If you use a document holder, place it at the same level as the monitor or inline with your monitor and keyboard.

There has been a lot of discussion about the proper term for more than one mouse—mice, mouses. I prefer vermin—it properly conveys the numbers of problems that arise from an improper mouse position and the over-dependence on the mouse.

• 8 •

Move It or Lose It
Workplace Exercises

by Heather Tick and Dwayne van Eerd

Always consult your healthcare professional before you embark on a new exercise program in order to make sure it is right for you.

Now that your workstation is all set up, it is time to move.

Neck Stretches

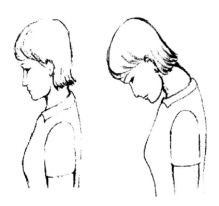

Sitting in a chair, begin by sitting tall with your head in a neutral position and eyes forward. Roll your head forward, tucking your chin toward your chest until you feel a stretch at the back of your neck or upper back. Hold the stretch for approx. 30 seconds.

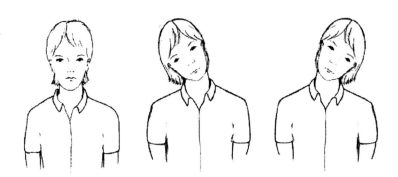

Sitting straight in a chair, with your head in a neutral position, look forward. Gently bring your ear to your shoulder without turning your head or lifting your shoulder until you feel a stretch. Hold the stretch for approx. 30 seconds, then repeat the other side.

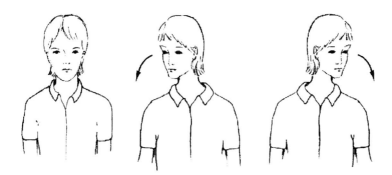

Sit straight in a chair, with your head in a neutral position. Without moving your chest or upper back, turn your head approximately 45 degrees to the right. Gently look down without turning or tilting your head until you feel a stretch. Hold the stretch for approx. 30 seconds, then repeat the other side.

Even with the best ergonomic equipment and proper set-up it is important to move around. Our bodies are not designed to remain static for long periods of time. Static positions put a steady load on our bodies: movement helps to reduce that load by having us use different muscle groups. It is recommended that you get up and move around at least once every hour during the entire workday. It is more important to move when you are under stress (i.e. deadlines). Studies have shown that you are more efficient when you take time to stretch. Be sure to do different tasks throughout the day. If you have a variety of tasks to complete, organize your day to switch tasks around throughout the day. At least a five-minute break every hour is recommended. Getting up and walking about (even just walking around your chair!) is one way to take a break. Stretching at your desk can also be helpful. The stretches pictured in this chapter are a basic set with which to begin.

Once you have developed symptoms or been diagnosed with an injury you should do these stretches once an hour at work, and several times outside of work.

Forearm Stretches

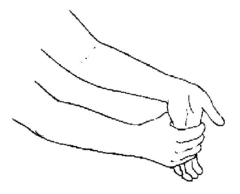

Without raising your shoulder, hold your arm out in front of you with your palm facing up and your albow slightly bent. Using your other hand, gently pull back on the palm of your hand, bending at the wrist until you feel a stretch in your forearm. Hold the stretch for approx. 30 seconds, then repeat the other side.

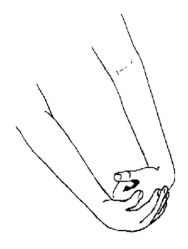

With your arms in front of your body, elbows slightly bent, make a fist with one hand and grasp it with the other. Now relax the fist but maintain it with your grasping hand. Gently pull the fist toward your body, bending at the wrist until you feel a stretch on the back of the forearm. Hold for approx. 30 seconds.

You should hold each stretch for 30 seconds. Count the number of breaths you take in 30 seconds and then time your stretch by the number of breaths (usually 8-10), since otherwise people tend to hold their breath while they stretch.

Spine & Shoulder Stretches

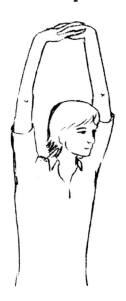

Clasp your hands together and raise them above your head. Turn your palms to the ceiling and raise your gaze to your hands. Hold for three breaths.

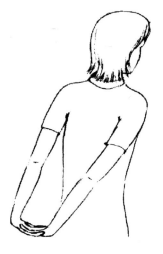

Clasp your hands behind your back. Turn your palms away from you, dn straighten your arms our behind you. Hold for three breaths, and feel the stretch across the front of your chest.

• 9 •
Exercises
for
Posture & Flexibility

Disclaimer: Consult your doctor, physical therapist or chiropractor regarding a safe exercise program for you. This is especially important if you are injured or have any medical conditions.

Core group of exercises

The spine is usually composed of 33 segments, 24 of which are moveable and form a graceful S shaped curve. The spine acts as a shock absorber for the body. When one part of the curve lacks flexibility, it is unable to take its fair share of the physical stresses. So the rest of the spine has to compensate. Muscle groups in the body are designed to complement and balance each other so that the push and pull can operate smoothly. The following exercises are designed to improve your posture by increasing the flexibility of your spine and the balance of your muscles.

Eagle arms

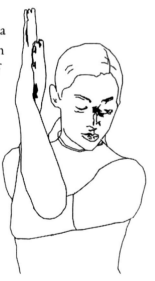

This is the arm portion of a Yoga pose called Eagle. Hold your arms out in front of you. Cross them over in front of you so the right elbow is on top of the left elbow. (They need to be crossed as tightly as you can get them.) Bend the forearms upwards and try to get your hands to face palm to palm. Hold for 30 seconds or longer. Feel the stretch across your back. If you need to intensify the stretch lift your elbows slightly. Repeat with the left elbow crossed on top of the right.

Bolster exercises

These exercises use an 8 x 24 inch yoga bolster which is firm and not very compressible. I like the ones stuffed with cotton. You can also roll a pillow lengthwise and wrap it in towels to get the right size bolster.

1) Sit on the ground with your feet out directly in front of you. Place the round end of the bolster behind you pressing into the back of your hips. Lie down onto the bolster, which now extends vertically from your hips to your head. You may need some support for your neck; use the smallest pillow or support that is comfortable. Extend your arms out to your side comfortably or fold them on your stomach. This exercise allows the pectoral muscles to relax fully. Begin with a few minutes in this position and then stay on it longer if this is comfortable. Some people like to fall asleep this way for a couple of hours. It helps with thoracic outlet syndrome (TOS) and carpal tunnel symptoms especially. (see Chapter 5)

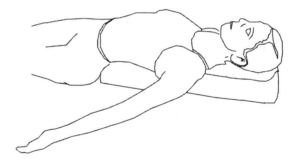

2) Sitting on the floor with your legs in front of you or cross legged, position the bolster horizontally so that when you lie back on top of the bolster, it is at the bottom of your shoulder blades. You may need a small pillow under your head if your spine is very stiff. If this hurts you neck, use a pillow. Raise your arms up over your head to intensify the stretch. Some people need to start very slowly with this exercise – only 15 seconds, and gradually build up

to stay in this pose for a few minutes. Breathing may feel difficult at first and gets easier as you build flexibility. (People with osteoporosis or osteopenia should consult their doctor before doing this exercise and should start with a very small bolster or rolled up towel.)

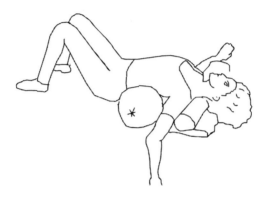

Scapular Retractions

This exercise is very subtle and can be easily done at the workstation. Sit or stand with your shoulders in a relaxed position. Imagine that there is a cord from the bottom tip of your right shoulder blade to your spine a few inches below that level. Now imagine that the cord is gently pulling your shoulder blade towards the spine and downwards. This is a very small movement as the shoulder blade slides downwards and inwards. Hold for a few seconds and repeat 5 times. Repeat on the left.

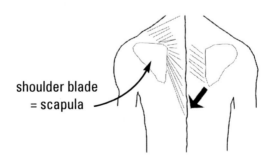

shoulder blade
= scapula

Shoulder Shrug

With your arms hanging at your side, raise your shoulders up towards your ears. Exaggerate the movement so you can feel tension in the muscles. Hold that position for 15 seconds then take a big breath in and as you breath out relax your shoulders downwards. This is a good way to remind you of the proper shoulder position because many of us tense our shoulders up as the day progresses.

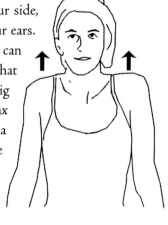

Cat Cow

This is also a Yoga exercise and it begins in the pose called Table. Get on your hands and knees with your hands directly below your shoulders and knees below your hips. Take a breath inwards as you curve your back upwards so that your head and your tailbone curve inwards. Exhale and arch your back so it becomes concave downwards. Continue for 15-20 breaths. This exercise lubricates the small joints of the spine and you can feel the difference in flexibility from the start to the finish of the exercise.

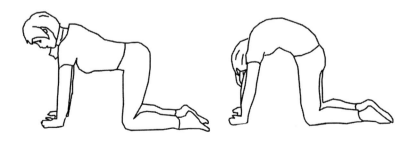

Chair twist

Sit facing forward in your chair. Cross your right knee over your left knee. Leaving your sit bones (the two bony protrusion you sit on) firmly planted on the seat, turn your torso to the right. Place your left elbow at the outside of your right knee and remain in the twisted position for 8 breaths. Now reverse to twist to the left. In the yoga tradition twists, are very important for improving mobility of the spine. What's more, they massage the internal organs and so improve bowel function. There are also twists for standing, lying or sitting on the floor. This one is useful since it can be done at work.

Side body stretches

1) *Seated*

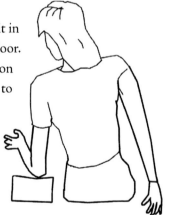

For this exercise you may either sit in a wide chair or cross-legged on the floor. Keep your sit bones planted firmly on the seat and lean to the right. Try to lean over far enough to rest your elbow on the floor or on the seat of the chair beside you. If you are unable to so use a phone book under your elbow until you can reach. Lean sideways from the waist and feel the increasing space between the top of your hipbone and the bottom of your ribs. Don't lean forward or lift your sit bones. Relax in this position and breathe (8 breaths). Then shift your elbow back an inch and hold for another 30 seconds. Repeat on the other side.

2) *Lying*

Lie down on your right side with your back at the very edge of your bed. Your buttocks should be right at the edge and your upper body should be at an angle towards the middle of the bed for stability. Drop your left leg back behind you so it drops down off the edge of the bed and stretches Tensor Fascia Lata (at the side of the hip) and Quadratus lumborum (at the side of your waist). Make sure your hips are lined up vertically and do not roll your hips to one side or the other. Hold for 10-15 breaths. Switch sides.

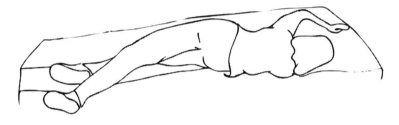

Piriformis Stretches

Hip and back stretches

Get on your hands and knees on the floor. Bring your right knee up between you hands. Now pivot your right leg so that the right foot is sticking out to the left and your leg is at an angle in front of you. Straighten your left leg behind you and slide it back as far as you can. Lower your upper body. You will now be lying down over your right leg. You should feel a stretch deep in your right buttock. Reverse sides for the left.

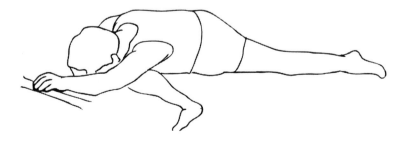

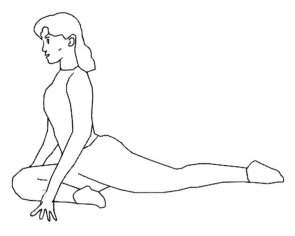

If this position is too much pressure on your knees then do the exercise standing behind a chair. Lift your right knee onto the back of the chair and pivot your right leg so that the foot moves to the left. (The entire lower leg may lie along the back of the chair if this is comfortable.) Lean forward towards the chair without bending at the waist. You can also do this stretch lying on your back with one leg in the air as pictured below. These are Piriformis muscle stretches. They are variations of the Yoga stretch called Pigeon.

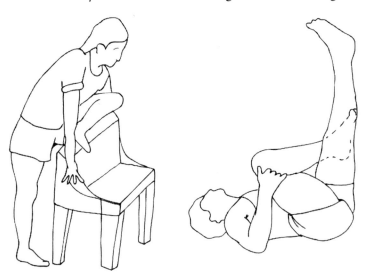

Overcoming Piriformis Syndrome

Piriformis syndrome is a very common cause of sciatica— pain down the back or side of the leg. Sciatica has in the past been thought to be caused by herniated or bulging vertebral discs in the back. In a recent study of 239 sciatica patients at Cedars Sinai, in Los Angeles, they found that only 3.4 % of them had herniated discs and 67.8% of them had piriformis syndrome.

Do the piriformis stretches to see if they relieve your back, hip or leg pain. If they do then do these stretches at least 3-4 times per day. You cannot do them too often. Hold the position for 1 minute at a time.

If you have piriformis syndrome, it is likely that your gluteal muscles on the same side are not working properly. Likely they become fatigued and stop functioning when you walk. Practice walking with your toes slightly facing inwards (in-toeing) rather than pointed out, ballerina style. This position will remind your gluteal muscles to stay engaged.

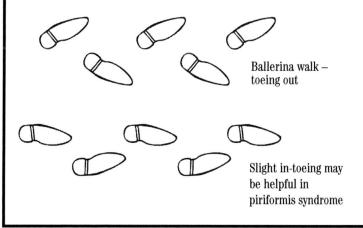

Ballerina walk – toeing out

Slight in-toeing may be helpful in piriformis syndrome

Front of the hip stretches

1) *Standing*

Stand with your back to the wall with your feet approximately one foot from the wall (distance will very with the height of the individual). Raise your right leg so the foot is flat against the wall and your lower leg is parallel to the floor. Tighten the buttocks and the thigh muscles of the right leg (similar to pushing against the wall). The purpose of this exercise is to open up the space at the front of the right hip. You should feel a straightening at the front of the hip. It is a very small movement. Do the same on the left. (This stretch was demonstrated to me by Gord Gow.)

2) *Lying*

Lie down on your back on your bed with your hips at the edge and your upper body at an angle towards the centre. Let the leg closest to the edge of the bed hang down and feel the stretch at the front of the hip. You may need to keep your knee straight (but not locked) in order to get the most effective stretch.

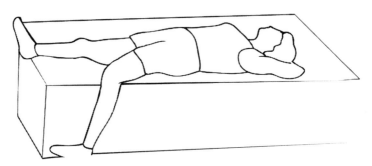

3) *Water jogging*

Using a floatation belt that clips around your waist (can be purchased from running stores or on the internet), you float without effort in deep water. By pushing the water with your arms and legs in running motions, you can achieve a high level of aerobic training as well as a resistance workout. If you are very injured or tired, make sure it is a warm water pool and begin very slowly with 1-2 minutes of "jogging" alternating with 5 minutes of rest. If you are more robust you can jog for longer and in a regular temperature pool. One leg at a time pushes the water forward as the other leg is carried back. The leg that goes back is stretching the psoas muscle on that side. Focus on that leg and make sure you do not arch your back as the leg goes back—that will more effectively stretch the psoas.

Calf muscles

While sitting at your desk put your feet flat on the floor. Raise your heels, put them back on the floor. Raise your toes and put them back on the floor. Repeat this cycle slowly, taking time to feel the stretches. Remember to breathe.

Swiss balls as chair substitutes

When you sit on one of these large inflated balls you have to use a lot of the small muscles in your back to keep adjusting your posture. Many of the patients we see for RSI also have back problems (even though some of them don't know it yet). We find that people's spines lose their flexibility from being in seated, static postures. The exercise balls can help this problem by encouraging movement of the spine and especially movement of the many small muscles that connect the spinal bones together. However, it is very unusual for the ball to function adequately as a full time chair substitute. Some people find them comfortable for a break at work, while reading and possibly also at the keyboard, if it is the right height. I often recommend them for home use while watching TV, reading or doing other seated activities.

Exercise balls are particularly useful for older people who may have developed problems with their balance due to stiffness of the spine. Use of the exercise ball must be done cautiously and with supervision and with the advice of a health care professional in order to avoid falling or sliding off the ball.

What to do if you get numbness while stretching

If you get numbness or tingling when you stretch, then gently come out of the stretch and breathe till the feeling returns to normal. After 30-60 seconds try the stretch again. Do a few repetitions and gradually over days you should be able to stretch for longer without numbness. Consult your healthcare professional if the numbness persists.

• 10 •
Healthy Habits

Rebecca is a 43 year old self employed consultant. She has suffered flagging health over the past 4 years. It began with a shoulder injury which would not heal fully despite many attempts at therapy. She could no longer play tennis or do her usual gym exercise routine. Two years ago she took up walking for exercise and began to get sore knees. Work was very pressured and for about 8 months all she did was work, eat fast foods and rarely exercise. Finally her husband insisted she see a doctor when he saw she was stiff getting out of bed in the morning.

Rebecca saw her family doctor who reassured her that there were no signs of arthritis in the blood. But he was at a loss to explain why she was so tired and in so much pain. He referred Rebecca to a rheumatologist. This doctor did even more blood tests and some x-rays. These tests did not give a diagnosis. He pressed on Rebeccas body on the 18 fibromyalgia points and since 16 of them elicited pain, he said she had fibromyalgia. He suggested Rebecca start to exercise again and he gave her a prescription for amitriptylline with instructions on how to increase the dose until her sleep improved.

Rebecca stayed with this routine for 2 months and felt no improvement. She came to my office afraid that she had ALS, or Lou Gerhig's disease (a serious and deteriorating neurologic disease where one loses the ability to move all the muscles of their body) and was fearful that she would lose her consulting business due to her ill health.

The physical examination of Rebecca revealed many ropey and tender muscles. Rebecca felt pain in almost any muscle that was firmly pressed. I discussed the difficulty in making a definitive diagnosis in the condition she was in and suggested a trial of therapy to see if she could improve. She began the IMS technique of using acupuncture needles, massage therapy, warm water exercise and postural exercises. She also ate healthy foods, used supplements to decrease inflammation and optimize healing and she controlled her work pressures by turning away consulting jobs. After 3 months, she was sleeping well, could go back to walking regularly and felt 40% less pain. She still wondered if she had fibromyalgia or myofascial pain.

After 3 months more, she no longer asked the question: Rebecca knew she was on her way back to good health. Her pain was reduced by 80%, she knew she would never sacrifice her health for her work again and she began to plan a ski vacation with her husband.

There are many things you can do for yourself, which will improve your general health, reduce your chances of getting injury when doing repetitive tasks and improve you rate of healing. The practice of Integrative Medicine has always been an integral part of our clinic philosophy. **Integrative Medicine** is a new term that encompasses the blending of both conventional allopathic (see glossary) and complementary alternative medicine (CAM) techniques. Integrative Medicine attempts to address the biological, psychological, social and spiritual aspects of health, healing and illness. It emphasizes a collaborative approach to patient care among practitioners of different disciplines. This Chapter will focus on lifestyle choices and self care practices.

Lifestyle Factors

Smoking—Stop it. Discontinuing smoking is the one factor over which you have control, that can most significantly reduce your risk of chronic and life threatening disease. In addition to all the other ways in which smoking damages your health it also starves your muscles of oxygen and makes it very difficult for your body to heal. There are so many bad things about smoking it's difficult to know where to begin. There are hundreds of carcinogens within tobacco smoke. But we all know about cancer, emphysema, chronic obstructive pulmonary disease (COPD), asthma and so forth. But did you know that smoking predisposes people to develop degenerative disc disease by a factor of almost triple as compared to non-smokers? Cigarette smoke contains a lot of tar. It is the tar and nicotine and some other nasty chemicals that clog up the small vessels (capillaries) that densely populate the border between the disc and the vertebrae. In fact, there is sort of a sandwich here, with the vertebrae and the disc being the bread and what's called a 'cartilage endplate' in between. It has been established that the disc, although completely devoid of any blood supply, does receive some nutrients via diffusion of these nutrients and gases from the blood supply within the vertebrae, across the cartilage endplate (a thick cartilage layer) and into and out of the disc itself. The chemicals within cigarette smoke cause a clogging of these small vessels and impair the diffusion of gases and nutrients-leading to further degenerative disease of the disc. The disc has no blood supply so the available oxygen is already somewhat precarious (2% oxygen in the disc compared to much higher oxygen concentrations in other tissues). Now, the disc cells are used to this environment but there's not a lot of room for error. Therefore, further impaired oxygen delivery imposed upon the disc and the cells within it, is part of what seems to tip things out of balance and increases the risk of degenerative disease.[4] Also, cigarette smokers fare far worse with many orthopaedic surgeries due to impaired circulation and poorer bony healing-this also occurs in the case of a fracture-smokers heal more slowly.

Exercise—A regular habit of 30-45 minutes of aerobic exercise at least 4 or 5 times per week helps with weight control, cardiovascular health, mood and energy levels. Walking is an excellent exercise and requires no equipment. Swimming, biking, running, and the use of exercise machines such as treadmills, rowing and elliptical trainers are also ways to get

---

[4] The physiology of the disc described by Mark Erwin DC, PhD.

your aerobic exercise. Even if you have sore arms and are limited in the ability to exercise them, doing lower body exercise will have a beneficial effect on the upper limbs due to the systemic changes in important body chemicals and hormones.

Nutrition—Eat lots of fruits and veggies, at least 5-10 servings per day. A portion is usually calculated as 1 cup of salad, 1/2 cup of cooked or dried fruits or 1 medium piece of raw fruit or vegetable such as an apple, carrot or orange. Juice should not count unless you puree the fresh fruits and veggies; ketchup is not a vegetable and neither are French fries because deep frying negates the value of the potato. Remember the computer saying—garbage in, garbage out. The same holds true for your body: if you want to be healthy, eat healthy fresh foods. With fruits and veggies—the more the better.

Supplements— If you are considering supplements be sure to consult with your physician, naturopath or nutritional consultant to ensure that you are taking the proper supplements and doses. Some supplements may be unhealthy for some individuals depending on their state of health. Three general qualities to look for in supplements: pharmaceutical grade production (ensures that what is on the label is in the pills), potency (based on the latest research regarding dosage needs, and whether the product dissolves in the stomach fast enough to be absorbed.[5]

Your body needs a constant supply of a variety of nutrients. The Merck Manual (a reference guide widely used by the medical community) cites 45 **essential nutrients** (ones we have to get from food or supplements because we can't make them ourselves). Other authorities cite higher numbers of nutrients. Roger Williams,

---

[5] *Comparitive Guide to Nutritional Supplements*, Lyle McWilliams.

(PhD), was a renowned University of Texas professor and researcher, who discovered pantothenic acid, Vit B5. His work also established that we all need different amounts of the specific nutrients based on our unique characteristics: that is, there is **individual variability** in our requirements. The published "Recommended Daily Allowances" for nutrients is based on how much we need in order to prevent disease and does not take into account how much is needed for optimal health or allow for individual variability. (*Nutrition Against Disease, Biochemical Individuality*, Roger Williams). Make sure you seek out good quality supplements. There have been recent independent studies done which looked at the contents of different vitamin preparations and how well absorbed the nutrients are.

B12—Recent studies indicate that even if blood tests are normal there is a benefit to additional B12 supplements for people in pain. The studies were done with injections of B12 given daily, because absorption for the gut is dependent on complex factors and may not be reliable. There is also sublingual (under the tongue) B12 which gets directly absorbed into the blood stream. Many people find this form sufficient, though injections are probably best. The form of B12 called methylcobalamine is the active form of the vitamin. Some people don't efficiently methylate B12 and folate to their active forms. Taking the methylated preparations is better for them.

Magnesium—is needed for muscles to relax. It can be helpful in painful conditions and for cramps, and it helps in the production of serotonin and melatonin. The chelated forms are best absorbed and utilized by the body. Too much magnesium gives you diarrhea and if you have kidney disease do not take extra magnesium before you consult your doctor.

Sleep masks—Research has shown that when our eyes are in total darkness when we sleep, our brains make more melatonin. This helps with the quality of our sleep but it also helps to establish the proper diurnal rhythm (day-night cycle) of hormones. One of these affected hormones is growth hormone which, in adults, helps healing.

Omega 3 Oils—Omega 3 oils are mostly found in fish and fish oils. Adequate amounts of these oils help to reduce inflammation in the body. They are being recommended to reduce pain and inflammatory conditions in the musculoskeletal system. A beneficial side effect of taking them may be reduction of cardiovascular risk (heart and stroke), improved mood, and reduced cancer rates. Use products that are not contaminated with heavy metals and other toxins.

Vit D and Calcium—Recent research has indicated that those who live in most areas of the northern hemisphere are vitamin D deficient. Childhood deficiency of Vitamin D causes rickets; long-term insufficiency of Vitamin D causes osteoporosis, raises the rates of certain cancers and autoimmune disorders. Vitamin D is the sunshine vitamin and is not found in fruits or vegetables. There is some in fish oils. International authorities have recognized the safety of high doses of vitamin D that were once considered toxic. Vitamin D3 is the form most usable by the body. Consult the latest recommendations about Vitamin D in the work of Reinhold Veith, PhD.

Vitamin C, sulphur, and magnesium for the production of collagen—Collagen is the tissue that the body uses to heal wounds. Adequate amounts are needed to make good collagen. The layers of collagen have cross-links and there will be fewer cross links if the nerve to the area is unhealthy. Smoking interferes with the production of good quality collagen.

Minerals—Recent research has shown that when we exercise and sweat, we lose not only sodium and chloride but a whole host of other minerals including calcium. Therefore it is important to replenish minerals using a good multimineral formulation after exercise.

Special Diets—There are books written on the topic of special diets for people who have ill health or pain. These include grain free, yeast free, nightshade free (tomato, potato, eggplant and pepper), high protein, vegan, and alkalinizing diets. Over the years I have seen successes with each of these regimens. Some people may have **Malabsorption Syndromes** which are a group of conditions that interfere with the absorption of nutrients from the stomach and intestines. There are many factors, which can cause an individual to be unable to benefit from the food they take in. A full discussion is beyond the scope of this book, but it is important to be aware that if you are not absorbing your nutrients, you may have a delay in healing. **Dysbiosis**—the abnormal growth of a virus, bacteria, parasite or fungus in a place it does not belong in the body— has become recognized in mainstream medicine in a few conditions—such as ulcers. In the gut, dysbiosis can interfere with absorption and cause an immune reaction and inflammation in the digestive tract. You need to see a professional for advice on how to try implementing these diets.

Celiac Disease is a condition involving malabsorption and inflammation that is getting more recognition as a cause of chronic pain and non-gastrointestinal health problems. Our knowledge of this disease is rapidly changing. People who are diagnosed with Celiac disease need a very specific diet. Celiac disease can be difficult to diagnose. If you are not getting better—ask for the test.

Alcohol—Drink in moderation only. If you need to drink every day, you have a problem. Alcohol is a toxin and it stresses your liver. Women are prone to liver disease with fewer drinks than men. It's not fair—but that's life. Wine, especially red wine, contains beneficial antioxidants.

Caffeine—There is a lot of conflicting research about caffeine. If you have muscle problems you should limit yourself to 1 cup per day at the most. Caffeine interferes with the movement of calcium in and out of your muscle cells. Caffeine also raises your blood sugar and jolts your adrenal glands (that is why it wakes you up). Because of this caffeine can also make you gain weight and tire out your adrenals if they are fatigued. Tea and chocolate have useful antioxidants and coffee may also.

The Hormone Connection—This discussion about hormone balance touches on a controversial and rapidly changing area in medicine. There have been many books written recently on the subject by reputable physicians and other professionals. Become informed.

Throughout the practice I have noticed several recurring themes that have made me question the hormone connection to pain and recovery from pain. There has been a subgroup of pain patients at our clinic who have complaints about difficulty with sleep, premenstrual syndrome, abnormalities of periods, excessive stress over a long period of time, frequent infections, feeling too hot or cold, weight gain especially around the middle, sugar cravings and mood swings. Many of these symptoms can be associated with imbalances in the many different hormonal systems in the body. Traditional Medicine has usually been focused on the extremes of hormone imbalance—enough of a change to show up on the typical blood tests. By the time people are at this stage they have a hormonal imbalance that is severe. Recently, newer techniques have shown us that there are subtle descents into glandular hypo-(under active) and hyper-function (overactive). Some of these subtleties may only be seen on salivary testing that more closely reflects tissue levels of hormones that are available for immediate use instead of blood levels of circulating hormones which include storage forms that can't be used right away. Other times the testing may not take into account the changes that happen within an individual over time and just lump all their tests into the normal range. For example, the normal range for TSH (thyroid stimulating hormone) is 0.5 to 5.0 at many labs. (Usually a higher TSH means that the thyroid function is under active). If someone usually had a level of around 1 and is now at 5, that individual may not feel their best. They may feel their energy is low, they may be constipated, gaining weight and feel cold. But most practitioners would call them normal for thyroid function. They may also have been through a lot of recent stress or be a perimenopausal woman, low in progesterone, and this may affect how their cells use thyroid hormones. There is a complicated interaction between all the hormone systems—sex hormones, thyroid, insulin and adrenals. It is far too complex to be summarized in a paragraph in this book and many books have been written on these topics (see bibliography). Our physiologic response to stress is the same whether it is physical or emotional stress. Pain is a stressor and therefore has an impact on the hormonal balance through its effects on the adrenal glands. Suffice it to say that these factors are important and should be reviewed in any case where pain is persistent or unresponsive to treatments.

Cortisol—When we are stressed our adrenal glands secrete cortisol. After being in pain for a long time some individuals have low cortisol levels and this makes their recovery go more slowly. This can be checked by blood tests and there are vitamin preparations which are designed to nourish the adrenals.

Thyroid hormones (see above)—An underactive thyroid can give rise to muscle achiness and delayed healing. Appropriate testing and treatment is needed.

Melatonin—See the discussion regarding sleep.

Sex Hormones—Estrogen, progesterone, testosterone and DHEA are the major sex hormones. There is a lot of current focus on the balance of hormones rather than just their absolute level. Much more research is needed.

Growth Hormone—This is a growing area of interest and is still controversial within conventional medicine. The Healthy Aging literature has more information to offer on this.

Toxicity—We live in an increasingly polluted environment and many of the toxins have a very long life in the environment. Just because we have banned leaded gasoline and DDT does not mean that there is not lingering toxicity in the soil, air, vegetation or water supply. We have been very surprised to find high levels of of heavy metals such as lead and mercury in some of our patient population. It is too early to say how many are affected and what is the source of exposure. Much more further study is needed to sort out how significant a factor this will be. The patients tested so far have been the ones who have failed to improve as expected. Toxicity may prove to be another factor that interferes with healing. Lead and mercury are neurotoxins—toxic to the nerves. They also interfere with the function of muscle cells. A simple blood test will only indicate acute exposure—within a few weeks. After that the heavy metals are absorbed by tissues of the body and cannot be found in the blood.

Sleep—Make sure that you get enough sleep (7-8 hours per night on average for most people.) Sleep establishes the proper environment for healing and because we are always injuring ourselves a few fibers at a time, we also need to optimize our healing.

Sleep position—it is very important to sleep in a comfortable position that does not put the neck, back or limbs into awkward postures. A pillow that provides neck support is crucial. This means the pillow must come right down to the base of the neck and support the entire neck. The neck is like a suspension bridge and if there is a pillow supporting only the head then the muscles of the neck are unsupported and unable to rest. A pillow, which has a bump at the end, is useful because it supports the contour of the neck. There are many neck pillows on the market but it can be difficult to decide which will be comfortable for you unless you try them first. This can get expensive, so I advise that you experiment with a rolled up towel at the end of your pillow first. See if you can determine the size and firmness of the contour that is most comfortable for you. Then you may be able to decide which neck pillow will best suit you. The adjustable ones such as the buckwheat or water pillow provide the advantage of being flexible. The buckwheat pillow can be warmed in the microwave.

1. If you sleep on your **side** make certain the pillow comes right down on a diagonal in front of you. You can place a large body pillow in front of you to rest your arm on. It will also keep you from rolling over. Some people also like a pillow behind them to keep from tossing around.

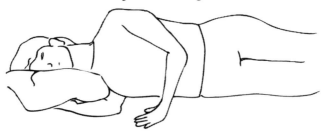

2. If you sleep on your **back** you may find that a pillow under your knees helps your low back. This is a good position to encourage the pectoral muscles to relax and allow the shoulder blades to slide towards the spine. If you have thoracic outlet problems you could benefit from sleeping on a slight incline with your head and shoulders elevated. You can purchase foam wedges for this purpose.

3. If you like to sleep on your **stomach** you are better off to break the habit because it is a strain on your neck. If you must be in this position, use a large body pillow in front of you and place it under half of your body. In that way you are not fully lying on your stomach and your neck can be in a more neutral position.

Physical Factors

Leg length—There is a lot of controversy over the significance of having one leg longer than the other. None of us is perfectly symmetrical. Most of us go through life with one longer leg without this ever becoming a factor in our comfort. However, when someone has pain in the back, neck, hips, legs or shoulders, it is often worthwhile checking the leg length. If there is 1/2 inch difference then a heel lift may help them to heal faster because the body will not have to make as many adjustments with each step. Try standing with one shoe on and one shoe off (shoe with a 1/2 inch heel) and see how it changes how your back feels when you walk. I have seen some patients where as little as 1/2 inch makes a difference in their ability to heal.

Eye dominance—Many of us have one eye that is dominant for reading: that is we read mainly with one of our eyes. This becomes important when we set up our workstation. If the left eye is dominant and the written work is on the right then you have to twist your neck to see it. ·

Alignment of joints such as knees, hips, elbows and wrists may determine which positions are comfortable for you and which may cause undue stress on the joints. These individual factors can be addressed by a physical therapist, chiropractor, osteopath or other therapist who is trained in the evaluation of body alignment.

Workstyle Choices

Ergonomics—The science and practice of designing or altering equipment and workstations to reduce injury, and improve comfort and productivity. See Chapters 6 and 7.

Stretches—Beneficial for workers who are in static postures and doing repetitive work. They improve circulation and muscle metabolism. See Chapter 8 and 9.

Work breaks—Taking breaks at work provides an ideal time for stretching. Taking a 5 minute break each hour makes people more productive. The stretches in Chapter 8 have been specifically grouped together as workplace upper body exercises.

Telephone Use—It seems impossible to hold a phone to your ear without tilting your head. Therefore if you need to use the phone for lengthy calls or use it repeatedly for frequent short calls, get a headset.

Voice Recognition Computer Software—Voice recognition technology has been helpful during the process of rehabilitation and return to work. It can be PART of an overall rehabilitation program for workers with RSI or MSD's. It should not be thought of as a total replacement for the keyboard and mouse, since workers with RSI are 11 times more likely to get vocal strain (RSI of the vocal chords) than people who use the Voice recognition for other reasons. It is best used for intermittent tasks to improve the productivity of the worker. See Appendix III for Singers Signs of Vocal Fatigue.

• 11 •
Other Occupations and Populations at Risk

by Dwayne van Eerd and Heather Tick

Graham was a 14 year old boy who wanted to be a computer programmer. He already had paying jobs doing website design. He did well in school and spent his spare time playing computer games. He also likes to compose using an electronic keyboard. He was not involved in any organized sports, and he rarely exercised. Around November, after exams, he began to develop very sore wrists. He did not tell his parents about it until his shoulders got so sore, he had trouble carrying his book pack. Graham hated vegetables, nuts and legumes but ate most other food groups if they were placed in from of him. If unsupervised he would reach for sweets and potato chips.

Graham started to see a physiotherapist who found him to be weak. He gave Graham a strengthening program using light weights. After the first week Graham had more pain and after three weeks his hands were turning red and clammy with exercise and when he typed. Alarmed, his parents had him stop the physiotherapy and come to the RSI Clinic.

Deborah is a 30 year old violinist who plays assistant first violin with the symphony. She has had pain in her right shoulder for many years but has always managed with massage and her exercise routine. She was almost unable to complete a concert recently and realized that she needed more intensive treatment for her shoulder which is held out to the side when she plays the violin. Her habits are all designed to optimize her health—she eats 10 servings of fruits and veggies each day, has fish 3 times a week, exercises daily, takes vitamin supplements and sleeps well.

So far this manual has focused on injuries that result from work involving computers. There has been a description of the risk factors associated with computer work as well as a suggestion of the type of prevention and treatment we recommend for resulting injuries/symptoms. There are a host of other jobs that have similar risk factors. Letter carriers, and sorters, garment workers, grocery checkers and cashiers all share similar risks and may present with similar patterns of injuries. Even going to school can place young people at risk.

Kids and RSI

We are seeing younger children with RSI injuries at our clinic. In Western societies, the children born in the late 80's are the first generation of kids who can't remember life without computers. In previous generations, children were more likely to walk to school, and spend hours outdoors playing with friends. For many reasons, children are less involved in unsupervised, spontaneous activities and they spend more time at the computer, playing video games or surfing the net. Some children are protected by being kinetic— always moving. Those are the kids who are up and down, may even climb up on their chair and never sit still. Some children combine video and computer activities with active physical lives involving sports, but some spend most of their time in sedentary activities, Galen Cranz's book "The Chair" is a very interesting chronicle of the relatively new tendency that we have for sitting in chairs and the disastrous results for our bodies. We see children who have begun prolonged sitting at young ages, and the muscles of their backs and abdomens have paid the price. The ones to worry about are those that hunch forward and spend hours, motionless, staring at screens. These children don't develop strong back and abdominal muscles, they have an exaggerated chin forward posture and often their shoulder blades "wing" out because the muscles are not strong enough to hold them down. Some children who play musical instruments are also prone to these injuries especially if they do not engage in sports that would strengthen their muscles.

Children are getting symptoms of RSI at young ages and more study is needed to clearly define the full scope of the problem. From the cases we have seen in the clinic, it seems that movement, likely protects the young and squirmy kids who fidget around a lot, hopping on and off their seats and even squat on them. Schools often have different sized children working at the same computer stations. Very little attention is being paid to teaching students safe computer work habits in the schools. There are some software programs designed for children, (offered to schools for free) that help reinforce proper habits.

It is crucially important to identify risk patterns in children, teach them proper techniques and encourage an active, healthy lifestyle.

Musician's injuries:

Another group of occupations (and often avocations) with known MSD (musculoskeletal disorder) risk factors are the performing arts. Visual artists, actors, writers (really computer workers!) and musicians are all potentially at risk for developing MSDs. At the RSI Clinic, we have seen individuals from all of these occupations. Most common among these occupations are musicians, perhaps not because they are more at risk but rather there are more musicians than other performing artists. This next section will present some information about musicians' injuries in this chapter (note that much of this can be adapted to other artistic occupations).

The risk factors are similar to that of computer workers: awkward or static prolonged postures, repetition, insufficient rest, deadlines, pressure to complete work, and muscle forces. Since the risk factors are almost identical the types of injuries sustained by musicians can be found in the earlier chapters of this book. With respect to MSDs there are no specific injuries related to being a musician. There are, however some non-MSD injuries specific to musicians such as the contact dermatitis a violinist may get from the violin rubbing against the skin of the neck, and certain lip injuries that trumpet (and other brass and wind) players may get.

Hearing loss is another specific disorder that can affect musicians who do not take the proper precautionary steps.

For MSDs in musicians, prevention and treatment are based on the same principles as mentioned previously for other occupations. The concept of proper posture, rest breaks, variety of tasks, good general health, diet/nutrition, and exercise all apply. In fact, proper posture, rest breaks and variety may be even more important for musicians. One reason why these risk factors are more important to musicians lies in the psychosocial demands of the occupation. If we think about typical computer workers, they often complete the tasks of their job under pressure of deadlines— or external pressures. Musicians may also perform work or practice with external pressures such as deadlines but often they work with internal pressures (i.e. they place demands on themselves). Many computer workers also put great demands on themselves, which can lead to injury. These internal pressures can lead to establishing practice (and playing) schedules that are too demanding both physically and mentally. Sometimes a side affect of internal and external pressures causes a musician to be so focused that they forget to take breaks. These pressures, and the habits that result, may be further compounded by additional temporary jobs or permanent employment (the dreaded but necessary "day job"). This is especially problematic if the day job involves computers or other static postures plus repetition. The time constraints that can be caused by the "day job" can also lead to more intense practicing with fewer breaks. In fact, as with computer work, taking more frequent breaks can actually help make the practicing more effective— quality versus quantity appears to be the key.

So, what do we recommend about the prevention and treatment of musicians' playing-related MSDs? Essentially the same principles established in the previous chapters of this handbook apply. However, an understanding of the unique physical demands of an instrument as well as the internal pressures inherent in the occupation is important. Paramount in this is the understanding that asking someone to stop playing is identical to asking someone to stop working. In situations of self-employment (musician or otherwise) the health professional must be sensitive to the need to keep working. For a musician to stop playing and practicing not only means a period of no work (and therefore no income) but because the level of performing ability can quickly be affected by the lack of playing/practice, the period off of work can be extended. This potential extended time off work can be very stressful and financially difficult. The musician and the health professional must work together to determine how to meet treatment goals with a minimum of disruption to playing and practicing.

The unique physical demands of different instruments and the postural and repetition demands are important to understand. A violist once mentioned the frustration of seeing many health professionals who did not understand her instrument and how it was played. This was most obvious in the case of one question she was asked by a health professional: "why don't you play left handed for a while until the symptoms subside?"

A requirement for optimal understanding of the interaction between musician and instrument is some assessment and treatment which involves playing the instrument. Just as the posture of a person at a computer workstation needs to be addressed so do the postural habits of the musician while playing their instrument. This is best done over a number of sessions so that change can be guided and observed.

An understanding of the demands posed by playing an instrument plus the principles of treatment and prevention noted in other chapters can result in effective resolution of MSDs.

Summary

The risk factors for musicians (and other performing artists) are similar to that of computer workers. The types of MSDs are identical to that of computer workers and the same treatment and prevention principles apply. As with computer workers, it is important to address the postural and muscle force issues that are specific to the instrument that is being played.

When Graham came to the RSI Clinic, he was examined and the most notable problem was his posture. His shoulders were rounded and his head hung forward when he was told to stand up straight. He had tight muscles in his neck and shoulders, in the front of his chest and in his arms and forearms. His hands turned red and clammy with the limited movement involved in the examination.

After examining Graham, I sat with him and his parents and discussed the possibilities for Graham. Many of the problems Graham presented with could be improved and even fixed. However, his desired long and short-term goals involve doing computer work all the time. I explained that we could work through the process of helping Graham to heal and improve his present symptoms, but I could not guarantee that he would be able to do as much keyboard work as he hoped. I could not predict the future. Everyone has a different capacity for repetitive work and we would have to reassess the situation as it unfolded.

Graham was instructed in proper diet and was given a regimen of supplements including fish oil and a multiple vitamin and mineral supplement. He was given postural and stretching exercises and taught how to set up his workstation properly. He was told he could not do any computer work for now. He was to walk for an hour 5 days a week for aerobic fitness. He worked with a massage therapist and physiotherapist. He tried a few sessions of Intramuscular Stimulation. He could see the dramatic effects of the technique but he did not like the therapy. He took a break from the needle technique after 3 sessions and continued it later when the massage therapist told him he needed another session to help loosen up some specific muscles.

After 6 weeks, Graham's hands no longer turned red with activity. He was enjoying the swimming class that his parents enrolled him in. His hands were not sore anymore. His activities were now increased to include a gradual return to computer work.

Graham continued with his therapists. The increase in computer work is slow but steady. If he overdoes it he can feel the pain return. Once he really overdid it and his hands got red again. He initially panicked, but was relieved when the symptom went away after a week of following his prescribed routine.

Graham is now able to do 4 hours a day in keyboarding. He feels confident that he will be able to increase this if he goes slowly. He also has gotten more efficient with his work—working things out in his head before he types them. He has decided to explore his love of music without using the electronic keyboard.

Deborah came for treatment after she decided to take some time off work. She feared being unable to finish a concert and urgently wanted to find solutions. When examined it was found that her right shoulder blade was not in the proper position but had slid too far forward, leaving the muscles between the shoulder blade and the spine overstretched. Other muscles around her shoulder blade were over tightened, putting traction on the shoulder blade and keeping it from moving smoothly. Essentially, every time she moved her left shoulder, her muscles were having a tug-of-war with each other. It was no wonder that she was having trouble.

Treatment focused on releasing the tight muscles and teaching her exercises to stretch those particular muscles. Deborah had to re-learn the proper position for her right shoulder blade and to recognize when it was out *of position. She brought her violin to many sessions so she could ensure she developed methods of playing and keeping her shoulder where it belonged. She was also taught self management techniques to help her be able to release the tight muscles as soon as they arose. She was absent from the orchestra for about a month. She continues with self management techniques, uses massage therapy and occasional IMS treatments.*

• 12 •
Types of Treatment

RSI injuries are best treated by a team of therapists who have an understanding of chronic injury to the muscles and a comprehensive, multidisciplinary approach. The current model of rehabilitation dictates a schedule for recovery that is more appropriate to acute injury (such as a sudden accident) rather than chronically derived injuries. The model, which was based on acute injuries, puts people with chronic injuries into strengthening programs before they are ready and often aggravates the original condition.

Often workers with RSI are very conscientious employees who have ignored early signs of injury because they had to get a job done. In addition, these workers often persevere in carrying out the tasks that caused their repetitive injury because they must continue to earn a living. The costs for workers and employers (time off work, reduced productivity, time away from leisure activities and family life etc.) associated with these injuries rises with the severity of the injury. In our experience with treating thousands of people with these injuries, early recognition and treatment is the most cost effective solution.

Acupuncture is the placement of fine needles into structures of the body for different purposes. Historical documents show that the practice of acupuncture has existed for at least 5000 years. The points are chosen on the basis of a system of medicine from the ancient times and does not relate to our scientific knowledge about how the organ systems work. Traditional Chinese Medicine and acupuncture can be helpful for many ailments.

Intramuscular Stimulation (GunnIMS©) is a 20th century advance in the use of the acupuncture needle for the treatment of myofascial disorders. Combining the ancient needle techniques of acupuncture with the modern scientific knowledge about medicine, C. Chan Gunn M.D., developed a form of treatment that addresses the root causes of these injuries. Dr. Gunn's theories were based on his observations of objective, visible, but subtle findings that can be seen on careful physical examination. GunnIMS© is the most effective and long lasting way of treating trigger points. (See Chapter 13 for more details)

Physiotherapy or physical therapy refer to the many different kinds of treatments that can be done by physiotherapists or physical therapists. Firstly it has to be done by someone who went to physio school. Each country, state or province will have rules about what is the "scope of practice" for physiotherapists. Some physiotherapy will involve many of the therapies listed and described below. Generally speaking the better quality therapy will take longer and require the full attention of the therapist (so they won't be treating several people at the same time.)

Manual therapy is a technique used by specially trained physiotherapists to improve joint alignment and function using hands on mobilization techniques. These techniques originated in Australia.

Chiropractic is a form of treatment that looks at the spine as being important in the evaluation of injuries in the body. Chiropractors focus on realignment of the vertebrae (the small segmental bones of the spine) and other bones. Chiropractic has the best results when it is combined with a therapy which treats the tight muscles that put pressure on the bones to keep them out of place. Many chiropractors will treat muscle tightness and prescribe exercise for weakness and muscle imbalance, as well as do adjustments.

Active Release Therapy is a term that the chiropractors have copyrighted. It is a massage technique involving deep pressure on muscle groups and has similarities to trigger point massage or stripping massage.

Massage therapy can be very useful for stimulating the circulation in muscles and relieving some of the tight bands or trigger points, and removing soft tissue barriers to the free movement of the muscles as they slide over each other. The most effective type of massage for myofascial disorders involves deep pressure on the tight areas. (May be called trigger point massage). You can learn to work on your own trigger points using massage techniques. There devices like tennis balls, specially designed canes or balls with bumps on them that can be used for this purpose.

Laser therapy (Low Intensity Light Therapy or Cold Laser) involves treatment with different wavelengths of light in order to improve healing in injured tissues. Research in laser therapy is ongoing and has to date shown that certain cell types are stimulated by particular wavelengths of light to produce growth factors in tissue. It increases blood flow. The best wavelengths are in the range of 690nm-840nm and the number of milliwatts is very important. We think the laser should be at least 75 Mw and we have successfully used 200Mw for many years.

Injections:

a) Trigger points can be injected with local anaesthetics and corticosteroids.

One can treat fewer TP's with injections as compared to IMS or dry needling. The substances injected may actually interfere with some of the mechanisms which cause healing in dry needling. There is a greater risk to injecting something using a cutting edge hypodermic needle (the type of needle used for all types of injections) and the acupuncture needles used in IMS can be used safely in many more areas of the body.

b) Botox is a substance derived from Botulism toxin. Botox blocks signals from the nerves to the muscles and stops the injected muscle from contracting. It is injected into muscles to weaken or paralyze them. This is the mechanism by which it relieves pain (and reduces wrinkles.) the effects may last up to 3 months. It can also be injected into the skin or just below it to block pain messages.

c) Prolotherapy uses dextrose (sugar) water to inject into tendons to cause irritation of the tendon. The subsequent inflammatory reaction tends to cause tightening of the tendon.

d) Facet joint injections can be used to definitively diagnose that the facet joint is the origin of the pain.

e) Nerve blocks can be used to diagnose and treat pain. Usually local anaesthetics , alone or in combination with steroids are used. Injections can also be made into the fluid filled area that is around the spine.

Osteopaths are a difficult group to generalize about since in different jurisdictions they have very different backgrounds. In the USA there are Osteopathic Medical schools which have the same status as allopathic (what we think of as conventional medicine) medical schools. In Canada physiotherapists and massage therapists can train at osteopath schools. And France and Britain have a different set of criteria for those who call themselves osteopaths. Generally, osteopathy is based on the theories of Andrew Taylor Still who was a frontier physician in Kansas, in the late 1800's. Osteopaths learn a very careful examination of spinal, and joint alignment and they use a variety of techniques to try to help their patients recover their optimal alignment. Their work is based on the principles that there are self-regulatory mechanisms in the body, that structure and function are interrelated.

Craniosacral therapy is one of the forms of therapy that is used by osteopaths and massage therapists in the USA and osteopathic trained therapists in Canada. This therapy is based on the work of Dr John Upledger form the mid-1970s. It is based on the principle that the fluid contained in the system that is made of the cranium (the bones of the head), the spinal column and the sacrum (the large bone at the base of the spine) has a natural pattern of ebb and flow. If some trauma interferes with this flow then symptoms ensue. They use gentle pressure on parts of that system to try to correct the abnormalities, which they can feel.

Movement therapies include Feldenkreis, Alexander, Mitzvah, and Bartinieff techniques. They are based on the principle that health can be restored through movement patterns. Many of us have had injuries without realizing how they change our movement pattern. We may not swing our arms equally; we may tilt slightly to one side. The movement therapies look at the patterns and try to improve awareness and restore optimal patterns.

Pilates is a form of exercise developed by Joseph Hubertus Pilates in the early 20th century. It was designed to promote flexibility and strength and has been very popular in the dance communities since the 1920s when Pilates moved to New York. Pilates Method focuses on core strength (the strength of the postural muscles of the abdomen and the upper back) keep the body well aligned. It helps develop body awareness, proper posture and alignment, while promoting flexibility and strength.

Yoga exercises and other eastern practices are ancient. Yoga, if it is well done with an instructor who understands injuries and knows how to modify the exercises appropriately, can offer an excellent blend of strengthening and toning. Research done comparing people who do yoga and conventional aerobic exercise with weights showed that the yoga group got fitter at the end of the study period. **Tai Chi** and **Qi Gong** are also moving meditations. They also offer a combination of stretch and strength. All these practices combine benefits for mind and body.

Exercise balls are sometimes used as an aid to stretching and strengthening. Some teachers use them for Pilates workouts. They add fun to exercise programs and can be very useful for stretching.

Wrist Splints may be useful in some of the MSDs (musculoskeletal disorders). Consult your therapist for your specific case. For CTS (Carpal Tunnel Syndrome) we usually recommend using splints at night to reduce numbness and tingling but suggest only intermittently use during the day. Splints which support the thumb for deQuervains' tenosynovitis can reduce pain and protect the thumb from excessive movement during the acute phase of the injury. Elbow splints for extensor and flexor tendonitis can also reduce symptoms. Care should be taken not to become over-reliant on splints since they can weaken muscles by not allowing you to use them.

Far Infrared Sauna is different from regular sauna in that it is not as hot and the source of heat is the wavelength of light called "far infrared". Infrared light penetrates deeply into the body and warms it. It has been used for detoxification (and many of those living in the industrialized world can benefit from the release of toxins) and many people find it relieves pain as well. From research on photopheresis of blood there is a growing understanding of the healing and regulatory influence that light has on our bodies. It makes sense when you think of the distant history of humans: we came into being as a species around the equator and would have been exposed to a great deal of light. So it should be no surprise that there are many functions in our bodies which are light responsive.As a side benefit people report that the far infrared sauna helps their complexion and even with some weight loss (when combined with exercise and diet).

Alpha Stim is a small electrical microcurrent machine that attaches to your earlobes. When turned on, it stimulates alpha waves in your brain — the same alpha waves you get from meditating. It helps with sleep, mood, anxiety and pain.

Muscles as the source of pain and the focus of treatment

Even when there is underlying arthritis or herniated discs, there is muscle tightening in addition. The muscle tightness is treatable and, in most cases, when the tight muscles are released there is some relief of the pain. Depending on the underlying condition, some of the pain may persist. Lengthening muscles reduces the traction on the associated structures such as nerves and tendons and increases the strength of muscles since they have their full length to generate force. Loosening muscles across a joint eases the pressure on the joint and reduces wear and tear.

• 13 •
Microsurgery with an Acupuncture Needle

People ask all the time: "What is the difference between IMS and acupuncture."

There is a world of difference and tremendous similarities between these two practices. Acupuncture uses fine needles according to the principles of Traditional Chinese Medicine (TCM), influencing energy pathways called meridians. Meridians are not visible, anatomical structures and western medicine doubted their existence until recent advances in functional MRI has been able to show that they do exist. (Professor Zang-Hee Cho, University of California, Irvine.) There are some newer systems of acupuncture combining anatomical principles of Western Medicine with TCM. These methods still use the same ancient acupuncture points and similar needle techniques.

C. Chan Gunn's system of using acupuncture needles is based on western medical science. It is called IMS (Intramuscular Stimulation) or Dry Needling. Dr. Gunn synthesized a system of treating musculoskeletal disorders using acupuncture needles to stimulate anatomical structures. He developed theories explaining why people developed painful conditions involving the musculoskeletal system. He explained that there is an underlying degenerative process of the spine by which we are all affected over time. There may be early changes even before the x-rays show the abnormalities. With these early changes come a subtle pressure on the nerves as they exit the spinal column. This pressure delays the healing processes in the muscles, which are fed by the affected nerves and makes the muscles hypersensitive (as explained by reknowned Harvard Professor of Physiology, Walter Cannon). This is called a myofascial disorder.

As we go about our day-to-day lives accumulating a series of small injuries, the healing process can't keep up and symptoms develop. Dr. Gunn's theories dictate that the muscles along the spine need to be released in order to optimize the function of the nerve and help the muscles to heal. Dr. Gunn described the physical signs that are evident when examining someone with a myofascial disorder. Professor John Bonica (Chairman of the University of Washington Pain Department and founder of the International Association for the Study of Pain), describes these signs in the comprehensive book, *Pain*. Dr. Gunn postulated that the dysfunction of nerves and the shortening of muscles cause increased stress on the joints leading to degenerative changes such as osteoarthritis. Salo, Bray, Erwin et al, have done research in the mouse model of osteoarthritis (OA) of the knee and demonstrated that most cases of OA of the knee were preceded by a loss of neurological control of the muscular forces controlling the knee. Further research is needed in humans but it may be possible to extrapolate that poorly functioning joints caused by weak, poorly coordinated muscles as the result of suboptimal neurological control may be a factor in developing OA. Tight muscles also cause pain by putting traction on other structures, such as tendons, nerves and blood vessels.

IMS involves the placement of acupuncture needles into locations in the muscles based on the physical examination of the muscles. Needles are precisely placed into injured and shortened parts of muscles called trigger points (TP's). There is an electrical impulse released from the muscle with needle insertion. The muscle may fasciculate or jump, or it may slowly cramp and then relax. In either case the result is muscle lengthening. Lengthening the muscles reduces pain by addressing the root cause of the problem—the shortened muscle.

When being treated with traditional acupuncture people often do not feel the needle insertion. The needles are left in place for approximately 20-30 minutes. With IMS the needle is being placed into the tender parts of the muscle and there is a deep ache within the muscle at most points that are properly treated. People can generally feel the release of the muscles immediately as the needles are inserted and left in place only until the muscle releases.

IMS points are chosen for the abnormality that exists in a particular part of particular muscles—the trigger points. Trigger points arise because the usual communication between the muscle and the nerve has been disrupted. It is like 2 old spouses who are not talking to each other very much. When the acupuncture needle is introduced it speaks the same language as the old couple and the nerve and the muscle each think the other started the conversation and they begin to communicate again. This and other factors encourage a healing process to begin.

With IMS the treatment points are chosen based on abnormal findings seen on the physical examination. In most cases there will be some immediate improvement in those physical signs. The treatment is done with precision and the results are often immediate.

Therefore, to summarize, IMS is the precise placement of needles to bring about an immediate physical change in an anatomical structure.

• 14 •
The Road To Recovery

Are we there yet?

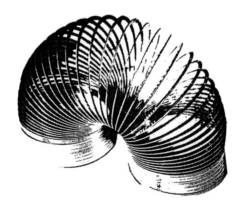

Celia is an English professor who has just written a book on Jane Austin. She had developed pain in her neck, shoulders and forearms three months ago but could not spare the time to limit her activities or to see the doctor. Now during the summer break she has had time to look after herself. She is diagnosed with RSI and begins a twice a week treatment program consisting of the Intramuscular Stimulation technique of acupuncture, massage and physiotherapy. She has a home exercise program and she avoids all typing and writing.

As September approaches, Celia wants to know how to safely incorporate writing and typing back into her activities. She tells the doctor that she has tried to type a little and can type for 15 minutes before her arms get sore.

It is decided that Celia should try to type for 12 minutes each hour at 9am, 10am, 1pm and 2pm. Celia does this for three days and notices that each day she is experiencing more pain. She reduces her typing to 3 sessions per day and is able to sustain this without increased pain. Celia continues this pace and after 4 weeks can re-introduce the fourth session of typing each day.

This seems like a slow and painstaking effort, but it is better to work slowly towards a successful work re-entry rather than hurry the process and result in relapse. The process requires frequent monitoring.

Frances is a 45 year old woman who has worked on a production line for the past 25 years. She works at a food processing plant doing a variety of tasks all of which are highly repetitive and require force. She had had aching in her arms, shoulders, upper back and sometimes lower back over the years, depending on which part of the production line she worked. Some of the work rooms were "cold" rooms so the food would not spoil. She was having more pain in her shoulders and her arms were becoming red and painful and sometimes she would lose feeling in her fingers after weeks in the cold room.

Finally Frances spoke to her union steward since she was having trouble reaching up to comb her hair, was dropping things because she could not feel them and could not open a jam jar on her own. A Workers Compensation form was filed and Frances was referred for therapy. When first assessed her shoulders were squared off and hiked up close to her ears. She looked as though she was wearing football shoulder pads! She could not put them down. Her hands and forearms were red and cold to touch. All her shoulder muscle patterns of movement for her shoulders were abnormal—the muscles were working in the wrong sequence.

Frances' therapy involved IMS, laser, massage and physiotherapy which had to re-teach her how to release her shoulders and how to use her shoulder muscles in movement. After months of therapy, she was ready to return to work for half days with no repetitive activity and no cold temperatures. Initially she had trouble meeting her job requirements for 4 hours, but gradually found she was stronger and able to get through her workday without making her pain worse. Her hands still turned red or white if they got cold—even walking down the dairy aisle at the supermarket caused this.

Frances is still working modified duties and hours and is the union is negotiating with the employer and Workers' Compensation about ways to increase her hours and productivity.

Some of the most difficult questions I am asked are about the time it will take someone to heal. Healing is a complex process involving tissue repair, re-establishing optimal patterns of muscle use, and achieving a balance of how much repetitive activity can be tolerated.

We are all familiar with the waxing and waning of symptoms. Chronic myofascial injuries (such as chronic low back, neck, forearm and rotator cuff injuries) can be especially frustrating to deal with because they do not follow a steady linear progression of healing. The analogy I like is the slinky. At every turn of the slinky there is an up and a down phase—in the same way that we all have good and bad days whether we are injured or not. The important thing to look at is the direction of the slinky—is it going upstairs, staying level or going downstairs. (Someone once pointed out to me that slinkies don't go upstairs and I responded that they were lacking imagination. According to scientific principles slinkies could go up the stairs if you put in enough energy.) It is often tempting to get caught up in the daily ups and downs, but what is more useful is to look past these variations and see the general trend on a longer term basis.

Treating these injuries likewise has a fluctuating course. When dealing with the work related musculoskeletal disorders (also called RSI) it is best overall for an injured person to try to maintain their work or activity level while undergoing treatment. This means, however that they will be partaking in activities that are known to injure them. Attempts should be made to modify the activities to make them less damaging—proper ergonomics, frequent stretch breaks during the work day, pace of work to reduce time pressures, varying the activities so not all of them are repetitive. For athletes and musicians involved in repetitive activities similar advice holds—vary activities, rest and stretch. It is important to keep the slinky in mind so that the injured worker doesn't get discouraged by the ups and downs, and yet is mindful of their overall improvement or deterioration. If the slinky starts to go downhill then the treatment approach needs to be re-evaluated.

• 15 •
Epilogue
Healing is a complex process

All too often these days I am faced with the dilemma of telling a patient, who is feeling ill, that there is good news and bad news. The good news is that all the tests in my conventional medical repertoire are normal; the bad news is that, I therefore don't know what is wrong with them. We are seeing more chronic illness, or perhaps it is better called "unwellness". The complaints are usually vague and nonspecific—that is not relating to any one specific disease entity. They don't have the chest pain of a heart attack, or the cough of pneumonia. But they feel tired, have aches and pains in a variety of locations and symptoms may shift through the days or weeks. Pain, weight gain, sleep disturbances, and a lack of the usual mental clarity are common complaints. But when all the tests come back normal there is little that conventional medicine has to offer. Sleeping pills, diet pills, pain pills all have their risks and side effects and under the conditions of a "non-disease" the risks usually outweigh the benefits.

There is a growing body of medical literature that is beginning to address these conditions. With the mapping of the genome (the genetic make up of human beings) there is growing understanding of the genetic diversity. Each of us inherits a set of genes that govern our bodies' functions and some of us will have genes that code for specific diseases. Some of these diseases will inevitably express themselves in our lives like Down syndrome or sickle cell anemia. Genes can acquire mutations which trigger such diseases as cancer and in other cases the gene only becomes a factor in health when we are under some kind of stress—physical or emotional. These stressors change the biochemistry of the body. We now know that our neurotransmitters (once thought only to allow nerve cells to communicate with each other and confined mainly to the nervous system and brain function) are available for communication with tissues throughout the body. Certain of our white blood cells (responsible for immune function) have receptor sites for all known neurotransmitters. Even more astounding, these white cells can actually produce neurotransmitters under stressful conditions. This means that our brain and our immune system have 2-way communication in an instant. Add to this that the gut has as many nerve cells in it as a small mammal's brain; that the heart has its own brain of 40,000 neurons and puts out an electromagnetic field that extends for 8 feet around the body and it becomes apparent that we have long underestimated the connectedness of the body-mind. Medicine has become sub-specialized and focused on ever-smaller fragments and sometimes we forget that all these parts are connected in an integrated human being.

It is important to look at the connections between the systems in order to understand the vague and often chronic slide into ill health that begins with feeling unwell and having no test to prove it. In practical terms, sometimes patients present with all the symptoms of low thyroid—they feel tired, cold and constipated, and gain weight easily. When the blood tests come back in the normal range no treatment is offered. By looking beyond normal tests into the connections of all the systems, there are treatments that can help to make people feel better. Proper nutrition is important; this includes eating the right foods and avoiding certain others. Some foods interfere with thyroid function and others may cause low level allergic reactions that stimulate the immune system in the wrong way and interfere with energy producing mechanisms. The addition of specific nutrients by way of supplements can also be helpful. Looking at the sources of stress on the body—lack of sleep or exercise, emotional stress—can also give some helpful clues.

Western medicine has focused on cause and effect of disease in a mechanistic way and hasn't embraced the interconnectedness of some of these symptom complexes. If, for example, the above patient also presents with palpitations then they would get bloodwork by their GP, they may get a bowel investigation by a stomach specialist and a heart exam by a cardiologist. Though I feel that these investigations are needed, they are designed to look for disease rather than distrubed function and often do not provide an answer. The body has a natural inclination to heal itself and many subtle factors can interfere with this process. It takes a more holistic process of evaluation to address unwellness that is not caused by a disease and uncover the factors that are interfering with the natural process of healing.

Sir William Osler, a reknowned physician in the early 1900's, whose legacies are still an integral part of our system of medical education once said:"If you listen carefully to the patient, they will tell you the diagnosis." In medical school I was taught that a proper assessment consisted of the history (getting the patient to tell you his or her story), physical (examining the patient), and special tests (blood work, x-rays, MRI etc) in third place. Over the past 20 years there have been increasing time pressures that have been placed on physicians. Studies show that the average patient visit to a primary care physician takes seven minutes and the physician interrupts 18 seconds after the patient begins to speak. This leaves little time for the history and physical and places more emphasis on the special tests.

Medicine needs to learn to balance the miracles of high tech, compartmentalized evaluations with the art of listening carefully. This is where healing begins.

Appendix I
"It's All in Your Everything"
by Mark Gilbert M.D.

At the end of one of the Mind-Body Group sessions run at our clinic, a patient with a severe and chronic back pain disorder sat up and exclaimed that "they always say 'it's all in your head.'" She was commenting on the countless physicians over the years who had inferred that because she had no physical findings or positive diagnostic tests she must be manufacturing her pain through her belief systems. At that point, another patient stood up and echoed what the group had learned—"No, it's all in your everything!" he said. What the group had come to understand by the statement "it's all in your everything" is that pain is now understood by science to be a concept shaped by every part of your being.

Now imagine that 'being' is by nature a complex organism that is made up of trillions of electrochemical and chemical reactions, which occur every millisecond of your life. You may fantasize this as a sophisticated virtual space exploration. Like the NASA space program, billions of space shuttle missions are sent out through your blood stream to find space stations in your body to "dock" with. Every space shuttle has its own configuration of a docking platform, and when it finds the exact locking fit with a space station somewhere in your brain, heart, liver, immune system or anywhere else in the body's solar system—docking occurs. An electrical and or chemical reaction happens that creates change, reaction, and cellular processes. Now in the example of your body, unlike the NASA program, those space shuttles are all made up of pieces of messenger proteins that are sent into 'body space' by different functioning organ systems. The protein messengers are called cytokines when sent out by your immune system, neurotransmitters (NTMs) when sent by your nervous system, and hormones when sent by your glandular system. These cytokines, NTMs and hormones "cruise" your inner space, communicating messages to docking receptor sites. When a muscle is injured, fatigued by overwork or stressed in other ways, NMTs are released with alerting messages to your whole body that something is "not right." Communication reaches every system in microseconds, reaching every pore of your body instantaneously. When skeletal muscle has been overtaxed, NTMs' receptor interactions allow pain to be experienced (or not) through a coordinating sensory organ in the brain called the 'thalamus'- the great pain coordinator. Messages are sent there along sensory nerve highways. Directions from the thalamus cause other neurotransmitter to dock with inflammatory cytokines in the immune system—asking them to protect the muscle fibers and calling on the hormonal messengers to narrow blood vessels. This sequence then alerts other NTMs to mark the muscle as needing protection, therefore secreting other pain messenger NTMs. In summary your nervous, immune, and glandular systems work together in a dynamic relationship to communicate feedback on how to cope with the over exhausted muscle fibers in question.

When the sensory messages reach your thalamus they are sent as NTMs to the thinking, motor and emotional parts of your brain. When they reach the front, middle and top of your brain cortex, these electrochemical reactions are organized into a series of symbolic thoughts that may, for example, say "my shoulder hurts...what a nuisance...I can't tolerate this...what's gone wrong?" The limbic lobe, the emotional centre of the brain, receives this message and responds with neurotransmitter messages of depression, anger, anxiety, and more. When the limbic NTMs of emotion are received by the preeminent frontal cortex (the higher thought-processing center) of the brain, they may be received and interpreted as "nuisance" visitors, and symbolic language thoughts like "this is terrible" will be received back by the limbic lobe as a signal that something "frightening" is happening In turn the limbic lobe will release depression and stress NTMs. Anxiety and agitation NTMs (norepinephrine, glycine and others) may dock with your muscle or nerve cells sending an alerting message back to the brain that "something terrible is happening." These messages, when announced through your body's communication mechanisms will send alerting notices to shut down the exhausted muscle fibers in question, making them taught, hyperirritable and with less blood flow. You begin to see the sophistication of the feedback cycle here...where "it's all in your everything".

In the days of the ancient Greek Philosopher, Hippocrates, before our scientific insights, there was nevertheless the intuitive belief that human organs systems could be healed and soothed through particular belief systems—using the mind to "soothe and heal the body." Traditional Eastern medical systems continued to focus on beliefs effecting illness and recovery, but in the Western world, scientific discoveries of the past 3 centuries made the philosophy that belief could help healing obsolete. The mind became seen as separate from the body, and therefore neither could influence each other. This naïve attitude held ground until a Harvard professor, Dr. Henry Beecher, made an important World War II discovery. Dr. Beecher noted this discovery after a fierce battle at the Anzio beachhead, when U.S. medics ran out of morphine to treat the war-wounded soldiers. These soldiers, suffering from horrific wounds and ready to go home to their loved ones, were made to believe that sterile saline injections actually contained morphine. A number of these soldiers felt significant pain relief. In fact, they did much better than post-surgical patients at the Harvard hospitals in Boston, who were treated with similar fake pain relievers, but without any war experience. Dr. Beecher came to believe that it was the soldier's knowledge that they were returning home to loved ones and out of harm's way that mediated their pain response to the sterile water. He called this effect "the placebo response"—placebo being a word taken from the sycophants or "flatterers" who sang Vespers on behalf of the deceased in the Middle Ages - as they were sent on safe passage to a better world. (Placebo is the Latin word for "we shall please".) People who wanted these prayers sung at the funeral were often charged enormous fees by the priests of the day—who did not likely share the same sense of loss as those in mourning. So the expression "placebo" came to stand as depreciatory code word for something that was insincere but nevertheless consoling. Since Dr. Beecher's studies there has been acceptance that about 30 to 35% of all treatment effects may be due to belief only. For this reason the so-called "double blind, placebo controlled" study has been used as the gold standard for all medication and other treatment trials. Ironically, the placebo response may be much higher than 35% (in fact some say as high as 70%) since these ethical trials require that the patient know that she/he has a 50% chance of being on a useless treatment. This alone can taint belief—and cause a "negative belief" or "nocebo" effect.

Remarkable scientific evidence of communicating messenger protein-parts in the body has been published in the most respected medical journals in the past 30 years. Perhaps none is more remarkable than the study done by Robert Ader at the University of Rochester. Dr. Ader was able to demonstrate that mice could be conditioned to alter their own immune systems by simply associating a sweet taste with a drug that suppressed their immunity. In order to get the mice to take the medication, Dr. Ader gave the mice a sweet tasting saccharine solution together with the highly toxic immune suppressant. After the mice associated the sweet taste with the toxic drug, they then were weaned off the toxic drug and given the sweet solution only. They still suppressed their immune systems! Thus the "belief" that they were given the toxic drug alone triggered an immune suppression. The more sophisticated enlarged human brain can not tell the difference between real and imagined symbols (just watch the emotional reaction of a child playing a virtual reality war game!) Dr. Ader's experiments later led to successful immune conditioning experiments in humans. Based on this and other research, it has been demonstrated that pain itself can be mediated, not only by the immune system, but also by gateways of belief systems, imagery, and suggestion.

This leads to the fact that pain patients have the opportunity to modulate their pain perception through a belief system as an adjuvant and powerful treatment option. After all, if NTMs from the cerebral "thinking" cortex send messages to other systems relaying that things are not as bad as was thought (and therefore not as needing of a distressed reaction,) than there is room for healing hope, pain dissipation, and immune enhancement.

Researchers in the United States have already proven this. Jon Kabat-Zin, the Director of Boston University's Stress Reduction Clinic for over 3 decades, has proven the benefits of pain control and belief using a specific technique called "mindfulness meditation." With this basic Tibetan meditation technique patients learn to be fully aware of their experiences in the present moment only, and without self-judgement. Being an objective observer to one's own thoughts, feelings and behaviours, one can get out of the battle with pain. The detachment from this distressing emotional struggle has been shown to decrease pain perception. Likewise, Dr. Herbert Benson, Director of the Mind-Body Medical Center at Harvard University, has shown that simple relaxation techniques (3 minutes just 3 times per day) of simple breathing exercises while focusing on a relaxing sound, image, prayer or tone can significantly improve health, diminish pain symptoms, and speed recovery. Hypnosis, a deep form of relaxation guided by a therapist's suggestions and story scripts, can also provide significant benefits in diminishing pain perception. So too can guided imagery, a technique by which one uses visualization or other sensory images to help promote relaxation, reduce stress and help the mind influence the body in positive ways.

Perhaps a more complex treatment approach to coping with pain, yet a highly successful one, is the help of supportive behavioural medicine or Mind-Body skills groups. A trained facilitator who helps to develop a healing community and teaches coping skills to deal with pain leads these groups. These skills need to include ways to re-think one's thoughts about self and life with perspective, truth, in a positive vein, and with a resilient attitude. Hope and purpose need to be re-established, relaxation skills taught and practiced, and the identification and expression of appropriate feelings fostered. The groups provide a safe place to establish spiritual connection, encourage journaling, and find time for appropriate humour, gentle exercise and proper nutrition. Mind-Body groups enable pain patients to reconnect with their community. They teach those suffering with chronic pain that they are in control of their life and need not be intimidated by pain.

It's not in your head. Your belief in hope, faith and a positive outcome despite pain, will be communicated to "your everything"— and given that, "your everything" will respond in kind.

Appendix II
Pain

Pain is a subjective experience (the person who has it is the only one who feels it). Hence all the problems associated with the assessment and treatment of people in pain. When pain results from a clear and visible cause—a cut, a broken bone, torn muscles—it is possible to get special tests to show clearly what is the problem or pathology. This testing will still not account for many aspects of the experience of pain, but at least there is some objective test that documents a problem. Sometimes people with very similar injuries will have very different pain experiences—some may have severe pain and require strong pain medication and some may need mild painkillers or none at all. It is sometimes seen as an indication of the person's character if they are perceived as having a "high" pain tolerance. But in fact we can't know what anyone else experiences when they are in pain—there are no objective measures.

Many doctors feel uncomfortable in treating pain once strong painkillers are required for longer that a few weeks. This is, in part, because of the fear of pain medication becoming addictive. Also there is unfortunately the possibility for abuse of these drugs and every doctor has encountered "drug seekers"—those who are trying to get drugs for sale to others or for their own recreational use. There are therefore strict rules and careful supervision by the Colleges or supervising bodies of the physicians. Doctors would like to avoid the hassle of scrutiny and therefore may decide not to treat chronic pain. There have also been recent legal complications for physicians who do treat pain, using narcotics. In a recent New York Times story (October 19, 2004 Sayyl Satel M.D., wrote about "Dr. Frank Fisher, a general practitioner in Shasta County, Calif., (who) was arrested by agents from the California state attorney general's office and charged with drug trafficking and murder. The arrest was based on records indicating that Dr. Fisher had been prescribing high doses of narcotic pain relievers to his patients, five of whom died. He lost his home and his medical practice and served five months in jail before it was discovered that the patients had died from accidents or from medical illnesses, not from the narcotics he prescribed."

With many cases of chronic pain it is not possible to have tests that indicate the cause of the pain. Often this is called neuropathic pain, but many other labels are used as well. When people seek drugs to alleviate pain that can't be "proven" by special tests, matters become even more complex. Recent research is beginning to explain the physical and chemical changes that happen to cause neuropathic pain and these developments will "legitimize" the condition. There are studies showing that a class of immune cells, called microglia, is involved in the development of chronic pain.

Analgesics attach to receptors on cells in the body. Recent studies have shown that not all individuals respond with the same amount of pain relief. There are genetic differences, which determine how much relief different people get from analgesics. This further complicates the pain treatment business since a standardized amount of drug does not guarantee a predictable response. In people who get sufficient relief from opioids, the benefits outweigh the risks and side-effects. For those who don't get good analgesic effects from opioids (probably on a genetic basis) the negative effects of the drugs prevail. As one patient with inadequate analgesic effect put it, "these drugs take away your soul". There is much research that remains to be done in the field of pain relief. Patients and doctors will benefit.

At our clinic we rarely need to use analgesics for myofascial injuries. We have found effective forms of therapy and we use non-drug interventions wherever possible.

Appendix III
Vocal Fatigue
Singer's Signs and Symptoms of Vocal Fatigue

Used with permission of Lois F. Singer

Lois F. Singer is the Director of the Voice Laboratory and Treatment Centre of Ontario. She is internationally recognized as an authority on vocal fatigue and has worked successfully with many of our patients.

Recognition of Vocal Fatigue can alleviate anxiety and help direct sufferers towards appropriate therapy. Investigations with otolaryngologists should be undertaken as well to rule out other problems that can give some of the same symptoms.

The following are **Singer's Signs and Symptoms of Vocal Fatigue.**

Signs and Symptoms of Vocal Fatigue in Speech Recognition Users.

Lois F. Singer, speech-language pathologist,
B.A., DSPA, Reg. CASLPO, S-LP(C),
Director Voice Laboratory and Treatment Centre of Ontario

Background

- A recent joint study with the Department of Rehabilitation Engineering at the University of Tennessee investigated the use of Speech Recognition as an alternative input device.

- A survey of **70 subjects** indicated that there was a statistically significant percentage of respondents using voice recognition software who are experiencing moderate to severe problems to their voice, viz. chronic hoarseness, sore throats, lowered pitch and even almost complete voice loss in as short as 5 continuous hours of usage.

Background

- Those likely to use voice recognition are people with severe repetitive strain injuries, Oesteo-arthritis or rheumatoid arthritis, are most vulnerable.

- From clinic studies of **30** additional patients at The Voice Laboratory and Treatment Centre of Ontario, a pattern of signs and symptoms of vocal fatigue and voice loss has emerged.

Case Example: Norway

- "When I got rsi in my arms, I was not able to understand the signals too late."
- "Aside of the rsi in my arms I got it as well in my leg up to the point I could not walk – I used a foot pedal to type with (!!!)."

- "Then I started to use the voice recognition program. Suddenly, one day after spending the whole day with the program, I felt some irritation in my throat.
- I relaxed for a week or so and thought that was it. But it came back."
- "When I realized that my throat and voice perhaps go in the same direction, I was terrified."

Case Example: South Africa

- "Has anyone seen cases of people who just can't use voice recognition safely? I used it for a short time (3hrs/day for a week) a month ago, and my throat's still sore!"

- "Perhaps some people can't use voice recognition even when they do everything right. Or just heal so slowly from voice injury that voice recognition isn't practical."

©2005 Lois F. Singer

Case Examples: New Zealand, Denver, San Francisco

- "My symptoms are a constant minor sore throat, that becomes painfully scratchy if I talk to people a lot, or talk to the computer, even a little. Symptoms have improved only slightly over the last many weeks."

- "I did everything correctly as far as I know: went to a voice teacher, did voice warm-ups, drank water, took breaks, etc."

- "Is there anything that speeds healing (besides the obvious rest)?"

©2005 Lois F. Singer

Singer's Signs and Symptoms of Vocal Fatigue for Speech Recognition Users

Phase 1: Onset

- Dry Throat
- Coughing Bouts
- Tight sore throat
- Neck muscles hurt
- Voice sounds breathy

- Difficulty making voice louder
- Voice sounds lower and lower
- Voice changes from high to low
- Error rate on SRP increases every 1/2 hour

©2005 Lois F. Singer

Singer's Signs and Symptoms of Vocal Fatigue for Speech Recognition Users

Phase 1: Action Required

- Drink water, suck candy, to increase flow of saliva
- Take breaks every 10-20 minutes
- Get up and walk around
- Hum softly
- Increase rest breaks

- Reduce number of sessions with speech recognition product
- Try to maintain higher pitched voice
- Alternate with keyboard, mouse and macro, if possible

©2005 Lois F. Singer

Singer's Signs and Symptoms of Vocal Fatigue for Speech Recognition Users

Phase 2: Progressive

- Same as Phase 1
- May get throat, ear and neck pains
- Increasingly difficult to make voice louder
- Voice breaks and cuts out
- Chronic hoarseness
- Error rate increases
- Can't sing
- People ask if you have a cold
- Recovery time from symptoms increases when off SRP, a few hours to day; reflects severity

©2005 Lois F. Singer

Singer's Signs and Symptoms of Vocal Fatigue for Speech Recognition Users

Phase 2: Action Required

- Discontinue use of SRP if symptoms persist after 1 week of rest from using the product
- Refer to physician and Speech-Language Pathologist experienced in vocal conditioning
- Check error patterns; i.e. number of errors in five minutes, location of errors, start, middle, end of words/sentence
- Check correction patterns; i.e. raising pitch, alter rate and volume

©2005 Lois F. Singer

Singer's Signs and Symptoms of Vocal Fatigue for Speech Recognition Users

Phase 3: Cumulative

- Severe voice fatigue
- Voice cuts out constantly
- Endurance is restricted to 5 minutes or less at any given time

- Voice range is 2 notes
- Voice is low, hoarse, barely audible, constant monotone and unreliable

©2005 Lois F. Singer

Singer's Signs and Symptoms of Vocal Fatigue for Speech Recognition Users

Phase 3: Action Required

- Refer to physician and Speech-Language Pathologist experienced in vocal conditioning

- Recovery may be partial and may span many months of intensive voice therapy

REST FROM SPEECH RECOGNITION PRODUCT WITHOUT THERAPY IS NOT SUFFICIENT

©2005 Lois F. Singer

Myths

- Myth
  - ◆ Drinking extra water during a session will solve voice problems.

- Reality
  - ◆ Drinking water is healthy and hydrates the body, but doesn't touch the larynx.
  - ◆ Anything in your mouth will cause salivation and lubricate the system.
  - ◆ If water is needed at the time, then your throat is probably irritated, and damage is being done over time.

©2005 Lois F. Singer

Myths

- Myth
  - ◆ Taking in additional air before each group of words will alleviate voice problems.

- Reality
  - ◆ Regulating airflow <u>in and out</u> is good standard practice for healthy voicing.
  - ◆ The issue is the use of the same muscles in the same repetitive way.

©2005 Lois F. Singer

Myths

- Myth
  - ◆ Esophageal Reflux is the cause of the voice problem.

- Reality
  - ◆ To protect the larynx, it should be treated aggressively.
  - ◆ It is an additional irritant, but usually not a sole cause.

Myths

- Myth
  - ◆ This problem is predominantly seen in hard-driving aggressive people.

- Reality
  - ◆ There is no hard evidence yet to establish personality type as a direct cause.

Tasks

- How are you going to use SRP?
  - ◆ Command macros
    - → Navigation
    - → Short codes, numbers

  - ◆ Dictating original text
    - → Letters, articles, books
    - → Each one has a different approach to voicing
    - → Each approach has different results

Recommendations

- Multi-modal Approach
  - ◆ Using systems that combine the use of mouse, keyboard and speech recognition.

  - ◆ SRP should only be considered as a helpful tool, not as a total replacement.

Recommendations

- Education
  - ◆ Users of SRP should be aware and conscious of the symptoms of Vocal Fatigue.

  - ◆ Users must recognize and act upon the symptoms pro-actively to prevent serious long term damage.

©2005 Lois F. Singer

Profile

- The profile that emerges is one of muscle fatigue and correlates to the over-use syndromes in RSI.

- The damage results from prolonged, intensive, repetitive use of muscle groups.

- The result is a gradual loss of power and strength of the muscles.

©2005 Lois F. Singer

Profile

- The larynx and supporting structures are muscle and cartilage, and are subject to the same restrictions as any other structure in the body.

- People vary in their ability to talk in a restricted fashion for extended periods of time.

Conclusion

- Ongoing research needs to be done to determine why persons with musculo-skeletal problems such as RSI, Rheumatoid and Oesteo-arthritis appear to be more vulnerable to voice problems when using speech recognition systems.

Reading List

Reading List

This list contains readings you might find helpful. It is not an exhaustive list. We do not necessarily agree with everything said in each publication, but they can help you educate yourself about the topic of repetitive strain injuries and the many factors involved in healing and general health.

Myofascial Disorders RSI Books and journal articles

Armstrong, T.J., Buckle, P., Fine, L.J., Hagberg, M., Jonsson, B., Kilbom, A., Kuorinka, I.A.A.,Silverstein, B.A., Sjogaard, G., & Viikari-Juntura, E.R.A."A conceptual model for work-related neck and upper-limb musculoskeletal disorders."

Anshel J.R., *Vision Health Management: Visual Ergonomics in the Workplace*

Erwin M.E., Inman R.D., "Notochord Cells Regulate Intervertebral Disc Chondrocyte Proteoglycan Production and Cell Proliferation."

Gilbert, M.D.,Tick, H., & VanEerd D., "*RSI*; What Is It, and What Are We Doing About It?."

Gunn, C.C., *The Gunn Approach to the Treatment of Chronic Pain*

Hagberg, M., Silverstein, B., Wells, R., Smith, R., Carayon, P., Hendrick, H., Perusse, M., and Kourinka, I. and Forcier, L. (eds). *Work-related Musculoskeletal Disorders (WMSD): A Handbook for Prevention*, 1995.

Higgs, P.E. & MacKinnon, S. E,"Repetitive Motion Injuries" *Annu. Rev Med 1995*

Horvath J., *Playing Less Hurt*

Iserhagen, S.J.,"Principles of Prevention for Cumulative Trauma"

Kome P., *Wounded Workers: The Politics of Musculoskeletal Injuries*

McGill S., *Low Back Disorders: Evidence Based Preventions and Rehabilitation*

Pascarelli and Quilter, *Repetitive Strain Injury: A Computer Users Guide*

Pruden, *Pain Erasure*

Putz-Anderson V., ed. [1988]. *Cumulative trauma disorders—A manual for musculoskeletal diseases of the upper limb.*

Simons and Travell, *Myofascial Pain and Dysfunction: The Trigger Point Manual*

Starlanyl D., Copeland M.E., *Fibromyalgia and Chronic Myofascial Pain: A Survival Manual*

Ergonomics and RSI Information Websites

www.cdc.gov/niosh/topics/ergonomics/
ergo.human.cornell.edu/
www.treatpain.ca
www.ergoweb.com/news/detail.cfm?id=562
www.humanics-es.com/
www.iwh.on.ca/
www.osha.gov/SLTC/ergonomics/index.html
http://web.princeton.edu/sites/ehs/healthsafetyguide/A4.htm

Mind-Body Medicine

Benson H, Klipper M, *The Relaxation Response*

Borysenko J *Milding the Body, Menging the Mind*

Childre D, *The Heartmath Solution*

Chopra D., *Perfect Health: the Complete Mind/Body Guide*

Dossey L, *The Extraordinary Healing Power of Ordinary Things*

Gilbert M.D., "Weaving Medicine Back Together: Mind–Body Medicine in the Twenty-First Century", *Journal of Complementary and Alternative Medicine.*

Gordon J., *Manifesto for a New Medicine*

Kabat-Zinn J., *Full Catastrophe Living: Using the Wisdom of Your Body and Mind to Face Stress, Pain and Illness*

Oz M. C., *Healing from the Heart*

Pert C., *Molecules of Emotion*

Remen R. N., *My Grandfather's Blessings, Kitchen Table Wisdom*

General Health

Blanchard K. Brill MA, *What Your Doctor May Not Tell You About Hypothyroidism*

Consortium of Academic Health Centers for Integrative Medicine; http://imconsortium.org/

Craig C, *Pilates on the Ball: A Comprehensive Bood and DVD Workout*

Ernst E, *The Desktop Guide to Complementary and Alternative Medicine*

Journal of Complementary and Alternative Medicine

Lee J., *What your Doctor May Not Tell You about Menopause*

Northrup C., *Womens' Bodies, Womens' Wisdom: Creating Physical and Emotional Health and Healing.*

Ornish D, Dr. Dean Ornish's Program for Reversing Heart Disease

Roizen M., Oz M., *You:The Owner's Manual: an Insider's Guide to the Body that Will Make You Healthier and Younger*

Weil, Andrew, *Natural Health, Natural Medicine: The Complete Guide to Wellness and Self-Care for Optimum Health*

Wood, E, *There's Always Help; There's Always Hope*

Glossary

Acupuncture – the use of very fine needles to stimulate certain structures in the body.

Acute pain – pain that is of recent origin

Allopathic Medicine – what we think of as conventional medicine taught to doctors in our current medical school system. Usually involves tests, drugs and procedures and is more concerned with treating disease that is already established.

Analgesics – pain killers

Anti-inflammatory –a class of drugs designed to reduce inflammation (see NSAIDs)

Botox – an injected substance used to block signals from the nerves to the muscles.

Bursa – a structure that is present around some joints which allows the layers of muscles to slide smoothly over each other when there is movement.

Bursitis – inflammatory condition of a bursa.

Carpal Tunnel – the half inch area at the inside of the wrist where the median vein artery and nerve pass from the forearm into the palmar surface of the hand.

Carpal Tunnel Syndrome – a condition where there is excessive pressure on the vein artery and nerve aw it passes the carpal tunnel. May cause numbness and tingling in the thumb, index, middle and half of the ring fingers.

Celiac Disease – is a condition which is characterized by a sensitivity to gluten. People with Celaic disease may show signs of it from early childhood and others seem to develop it in adulthood. Sometimes the symptoms relate to the bowel and sometimes to other systems in the body. It can be associated with pain anywhere in the body.

Chronic pain – pain lasting longer than 6 months (some authorities use 3 months)

Chronic regional pain syndrome – CRPS – chronic pain that is thought to be maintained by a malfunction of the Sympathetic nervous system

Craniosacral therapy – a very gentle technique of affecting tightness in deep structures of the body

CTD – same as RSI – cumulative trauma disorder

de Quervains' tenosynovitis – inflammation of the tendons that pass to the outside of the thumb

EMG – electromyography, a test where reading of the electrical output of muscles is measured – usually involves a needle and looks at small units of the muscle (see sEMG)

Ergonomics – the field of study that tries to find out what human bodies require from their work environment In order to work efficiently and safely without injury

Fibromyalgia – the painful condition defined as having the following criteria: a sleep disorder and eleven of eighteen specific points on the body that are tender. There should be upper and lower body, and right and left sided pain

Healing – the process by which there is improvement in an illness or condition. May not involve curing or fixing the problem.

IMS – also called dry needling. A technique using acupuncture needles to stimulate myofascial trigger points

Integrative Medicine – the latest in the terms used to describe the integrated use of multidisciplinary teams to prevent illness and treat disease. This has been called alternative medicine or complementary medicine in the past. These approaches to medicine focus on prevention and they pay attention to mind, body, and spirit.

Interscapular Muscles – the muscles between the shoulder blades. These muscles stabilize the shoulder blades or scapulae.

Intervetebral discs – These structures act like cushions between the vertebrae or spinal bones.

Irritable bowel – is often diagnosed when there are vague symptoms in the absence of disease. Symptoms may come and go, often related to food intolerance or dybiosis. Beware of treating a non-disease with drugs that can have serious side effects.

Laser therapy – the use of low intensity laser light to put energy into tissues and stimulate healing.

Mind body medicine – the growing field of medicine that integrates the treatment of the different systems of the body as well as psychological and spiritual aspects into the treatment of the whole person. A holistic approach to health care that recognizes the interconnectedness of all the systems of the human being and tries to take as many of these into account as possible when formulating an approach to curing illness.

Movement therapies – There are several schools of movement therapy. They all take the student back to an awareness of more efficient and basic patterns of movement.

Myofascial – affecting the muscles and supporting connective tissues, usually involves trigger points in muscles

MSD – musculoskeletal disorder, also called WMSD (work related muskuloskeletal disorder) in some literature. Means the same as RSI and is probably the best term to use when describing these injuries

Nerve conduction test – a test looking at the speed with which a nerve passes electrical current along its path. May be normal in the presence of nerve compression as long as the nerve is not dying yet.

Non steroidal anti-inflammatory (NSAIDs) – anti-inflammatory that is not a steroid; these usually also have some pain relieving effects in addition.

OOS – same as RSI Occupational overuse syndrome

Parasympathetic nervous system – the part of the autonomic nervous system that is responsible for the normal functioning of many of our internal organ systems. It is designed to be in balance with the sympathetic nervous system.

Piriformis Syndrome – This syndrome is usually caused by tightness of the muscle which is deep in the buttock. This muscle lies in very close contact with the sciatic nerve and can cause pressure on that nerve resulting in sciatica. Piriformis syndrome can mimic a herniated disc in the lumbar spine (also called a slipped or bulging disc).

Prolotherapy – an injection technique to tighten ligaments and tendons

Reflex sympathetic dystrophy – an older name for CRPS

Rotator cuff tendonitis – tendonitis of the rotator cuff tendons which are around the shoulder blade

Rotator cuff dysfunction – a more common condition where inflammation does not play a major role, but the rotator cuff muscles do not function efficiently

RSI – repetitive strain injury, an injury which occurs when most of the body is in a static posture and a few parts of the body are used to do the same or similar activities repeatedly

Sciatica – Pain down the back or side of the thigh and leg caused by pressure on the nerves of the low back. It has commonly been thought to be caused by pressure from the intervertebral discs, but recent studies have confirmed that piriformis synrome is more common.

SEMG – a test using surface electrode to examine the electrical activity of muscles. The test involves no needles and looks at the usage patterns of muscle functional units or large units of muscle.

Steroid – an anti-inflammatory drug that mimics the cortisol from our adrenal glands

Sympathetic nervous system – part of the autonomic nervous system responsible for the fight or flight reaction. It gets overstimulated when someone is anxious

Tenosynovitis – inflammation of a tendon sheath that has an extra layer of connective tissue called synovium

Tendon – the connective tissue that attaches muscle to bone

Tendonitis – inflammation of tendons. Sometimes the label is applied when there is only tenderness and no appreciable inflammation

Thoracic outlet syndrome – compression of the vein, artery and nerves as they pass through the thoracic outlet

Thoracic outlet – the area at the side of the neck where the veins, arteries and nerves can become compressed, usually by over tight muscles, but may also be by connective tissue bands or the presence of an extra cervical vertebrae.

Trigger points (TP's) – over contracted, injured areas of muscle

Trigger Point massage – a technique using very firm pressure in order to release TP's

Index